The Smallpox Eradication Saga

New Perspectives in South Asian History 33

The **New Perspectives in South Asian History** series publishes monographs and other writings on early modern, modern and contemporary history. The volumes in the series cover new ground across a broad spectrum of subjects such as cultural, environmental, medical, military and political history, and the histories of 'marginalised' groups. It includes fresh perspectives on more familiar fields as well as interdisciplinary and original work from all parts of South Asia. It welcomes historical contributions from sociology, anthropology and cultural studies.

The Smallpox Eradication Saga
An Insider's View

ISAO ARITA

Edited by
Alan Schnur
Masanobu Sugimoto

Foreword by
David L. Heymann

Orient BlackSwan

ORIENT BLACKSWAN PRIVATE LIMITED

Registered Office
3-6-752 Himayatnagar, Hyderabad 500 029 (A.P.), India
E-mail: centraloffice@orientblackswan.com

Other Offices
Bangalore, Bhopal, Bhubaneshwar, Chandigarh, Chennai, Ernakulam, Guwahati, Hyderabad, Jaipur, Kolkata, Lucknow, Mumbai, New Delhi, Noida, Patna

First Published 2010

ISBN 978 81 250 4095 8

Typeset by
OSDATA, Hyderabad 500 029
in Bembo (Aldine) 10.5/12.5

Maps cartographed by
Sangam Books (India) Private Limited, Hyderabad

Printed at
Aegean Offset, Greater Noida

Published by
Orient Blackswan Private Limited
1/24 Asaf Ali Road, New Delhi 110 002
E-mail: delhi@orientblackswan.com

For my wife, Shigeruko,
my daughers, Bara and Erika,
and in friendly memory of the programme families

Contents

Figures, Tables, Maps and Boxes

Foreword

David L. Heymann

It is hard to believe that as recently as 1967, the smallpox virus was killing an estimated 3 million people each year and leaving countless others scarred for life, often with such severe facial pockmarks and blinding corneal scars that even when they recovered from infection, they were shunned by society. Those who have not seen smallpox cannot know the fear that it caused in those who were ill, as well as among their families and friends.

The story of smallpox eradication is many stories rolled into one. It's a story not only of the fieldwork that led to the successful interruption of human-to-human transmission and the victory of eradication, but also of the dynamism of infectious diseases in nature, as one replaces or interacts with another. Sadly, it is also a story of the smallpox virus, perhaps even having fallen into the hands of those who are evil enough to deliberately cause harm. Isao Arita has described the fieldwork that led to eradication as few others could. He has shared a true insider's view of the programme in Geneva, where the activities were coordinated at the World Health Organization (WHO). And as Isao mentions more than once, in order to accomplish eradication, it took the courage to bend inflexible international bureaucracy, and at times to break the rules that were impeding success. But, at the same time, Isao used the experience and evidence base from his early years as a fieldworker in Liberia to tailor the programme activities to better ensure success.

I was fortunate to be one of the young international public health workers recruited by WHO to work in the smallpox eradication programme during the 1970s. For those of us who worked in the field under the guidance of Isao Arita, D. A. Henderson and their colleagues, little did we know at the start that the activities in which we were about to participate would lead to one of the world's greatest public health accomplishments. They were also to lead us to membership in a fraternity of public health workers that produced national and international leaders in public health during the latter part of the twentieth century. What better tribute to Isao and his co-workers. And what better lesson than that of the power of vaccines.

But smallpox eradication might not have happened if the drive of its leaders had waned before 1980. In 1981, just after smallpox eradication had been certified through the process Isao so clearly describes, a new infectious disease was first identified. That disease was AIDS, caused by HIV—a virus that surpasses smallpox in its end-stage virulence. In 1980, HIV was just beginning to amplify in transmission as it found its way from rural areas of sub-Saharan Africa where it had crossed the species barrier to humans, to urban areas where sexual promiscuity provided it with the unfortunate opportunity to spread. From these urban centres, international travel rapidly spread the virus throughout Africa and the world. One viral infectious disease, smallpox, was conquered, and another had taken its place.

Three years later, in 1984, a military recruit in the United States, unknown to be infected with HIV, was immunised with the smallpox vaccine. From this live virus vaccine he developed the condition generalised vaccinia, an AIDS-defining event that led to AIDS and death six months later. With up to 30 per cent of some adult populations infected with HIV in sub-Saharan Africa, and HIV infections throughout the world, the vaccine that was used to eradicate smallpox cannot now be safely used in HIV-infected populations. A window of opportunity to eradicate smallpox is now closed, but fortunately it closed only after the world was rid of smallpox. Isao and his colleagues took advantage of a window of opportunity as they led the world to eradication, without even knowing that the window was closing. The lesson for us all in this is this: do the best with what public health tools we have today because the window of opportunity may be closed tomorrow. It is good fortune that oral polio vaccines used for polio eradication can safely be used in HIV-infected children—the window of opportunity to eradicate that vicious virus remains open.

Even before HIV, though, it was known that the vaccines used to eradicate smallpox were imperfect. Though they produced solid immunity against smallpox infection in those who were successfully vaccinated, approximately one in every million vaccinated developed a neurological complication, and some died. But the risk of dying from the vaccine was much lower than dying from smallpox, so the risk-benefit analysis favoured smallpox eradication.

Once eradication had been certified, countries rapidly stopped smallpox vaccination: the risk-benefit ratio had changed, as the risk of death from vaccination had now become greater than the risk of death from infection. But as Isao points out, there are rumours that since eradication, the virus is not being exclusively held under maximum bio security in the two known and approved laboratories, but that it is also in the hands of those who might hope to use it for malicious purposes in a world where the population is no longer being vaccinated. Unthinkable as it is, the risk, and the risk-benefit ratio of smallpox vaccination, could one day change again.

I remember discussing this situation with Isao in the late 1990s, when WHO's member states requested that guidance for smallpox containment be updated and that smallpox vaccine stockpiles be reconstituted. I also remember discussing the polio situation with Isao when the polio virus began to spread and re-infect countries that had previously been polio free, stalling polio eradication activities in the early 2000s. The wisdom given then is the same as the wisdom that comes through in this book—the wisdom of a quiet and effective leader, with undying persistence to reach a goal.

The story of smallpox eradication is enshrined in the monument that stands at the entrance of WHO in Geneva: a partnership of nations that worked together to free the world of a dreaded disease; a story of success in public health, and of untiring leadership and devotion. That leadership and devotion are most clearly shown in the book that follows.

Prologue

The year 2009 marked the 150th anniversary of Charles Darwin's publication of *On the Origin of Species by Means of Natural Selection, or the Preservation of Favored Races in the Struggle for Life*. Accordingly, the media and the global scientific community have been discussing the evolution of biological species. Under the circumstances, I feel smallpox eradication may be defined as an initiative whereby human efforts successfully resulted in a dangerous pathogen's disappearance from the planet. The eradication of this disease resulted in improved human survival by removing the menace of the smallpox virus that had caused great suffering and a significant number of deaths throughout human history.

The history of smallpox eradication has been meticulously documented in a 1500-page encyclopaedic World Health Organization book, *Smallpox and its Eradication*, published in 1988.[1] I was one of the five authors of this large volume (nicknamed "The Big Red Book" from its cadmium red-coloured hard cover) that includes every aspect of the disease and the efforts of the smallpox eradication programme to rid the world of this scourge. Although proud of my contribution to this book, the one problem with it is that it is much too large for someone to easily read through it. Let me say that the "Big Red Book" is a valuable addition to a library of some institution, to provide an excellent source of reference information whenever someone has some queries or is researching a special subject.

Therefore, I felt it would be beneficial to write a shorter, more accessible book covering my personal experiences as a WHO medical officer when working for the smallpox eradication programme.

[1] F. Fenner, D. A. Henderson, I. Arita, Z. Jezek and L D. Ladnyi, *Smallpox and its Eradication* (Washington, D.C: World Health Organisation, 1988)

In the book, I have tried to describe how the WHO initiative was supported by tremendous human efforts, made by people from different cultures, races, nationalities and religions, and also by the unification of the global scientific community.

I participated in the WHO-led effort from 1962 to 1985, over a period of twenty-three years. It included the smallpox eradication preparatory phase from 1962 to 1966; an intensified smallpox eradication and certification phase, with WHO regular budget and international support, from 1967 to 1980; and the tedious work of developing preparedness to prevent the return of smallpox if it occurred, documenting the effort and sorting out historical records from 1981 to 1985. Thus, this book covers not only what happened during the period of the actual smallpox eradication programme on a global basis, but also what happened in the post-eradication era, including the treatment of remaining smallpox virus stocks, preparedness for bio terrorism and related research to sustain a smallpox free world. As a member of the WHO Smallpox Research Committee, I would like to point out that the last lot of activities could be termed work-in-progress and continue to this day.

In the book, I have also tried to judge my experiences objectively from the viewpoint of what lessons have been learnt, so that they may provide useful information to current and future generations in a narrative manner. Hopefully, the book will also help those readers without much experience in public health to read about smallpox eradication and understand how theories may be transferred to actual field operations. In this respect I was fortunate to have two of my smallpox eradication programme colleagues, Alan Schnur (originally a US Peace Corps volunteer and later WHO technical officer) and Masanobu Sugimoto (a research scientist of molecular biology in Japan). They helped edit the text as well as check technical accuracy of the contents.

I have named many of my smallpox programme colleagues in this book. However there were several others who, although not mentioned in this book contributed significantly to the events I describe. Since this book narrates my personal experience, I have had to limit the names mentioned to those with whom I had close personal contact during my work, both at the official as well as village level.

One last point I would like to make is that I, personally, feel that smallpox eradication could only have been achieved under WHO leadership and coordination. Needless to say, the functioning of any system depends very much upon the people who work in the system. Smallpox eradication was achieved using the WHO system to recruit and support dedicated and talented international personnel who worked successfully at all levels of the programme.

There are many books and reports which describe how smallpox eradication was successfully carried out. My hope is that this book will contribute to the existing literature in a broader sense, in understanding this unprecedented programme in human evolutionary development, or in the human ability of survival, as Darwin first discussed. In Japan, we have a proverb that says, "hearing a hundred times is not as effective as just one glance in person". I trust that the descriptions of my personal impressions while I was actively involved in the day to day running of the programme will serve to provide the reader with many glances into the programme, and how it succeeded in ridding the planet of smallpox.

Isao Arita

Acknowledgements

This book is largely based on my earlier book in Japanese, *Smallpox Eradication—Target Zero*, published in October 1979 by the Mainichi Press, the major newspaper in Japan. This was 30 years ago and I am particularly grateful to my co-workers in the World Health Organization Smallpox Eradication Unit for their assistance during the last phase of the programme. At the time I was extremely busy, but their help enabled me to prepare, say every weekend, the important note or aide memoir which served to coordinate the busy work plans at that time, and which finally became the valuable basis for this current publication. My heartfelt thanks to Joel G. Breman, Robert N. Evans, Alex I. Gromyko, Ron Hauge, Zdeno Jezek, James Magee, Jim L. Tulloch, John F. Wickett, Celia Sands and Susan Woolnough.

I continue to think of my old experience in smallpox eradication from the viewpoint of what happened during the active period of smallpox eradication, as well as what has been happening in the post-eradication era until now. In this respect, I have learnt a great deal about how to regard my own experience from a fresh point of view. Thus, I have been able to elaborate my experiences further, and this has enabled my writing this book. In this respect, I am deeply indebted to the many experts who have given me insightful information and advice. Unfortunately not all can be mentioned here, but I would like to specially thank Bruce Aylward, Seth Berkley, Julian Bilous, Anthony Burton, D. A. Henderson, David Heymann, Kazunobu Kojima, Svetlana Marennikova, Elizabeth Mason, Tatsuo Myamura, Andre Platinga, Robert Scherpbier and Rudolf Tangermann.

For the practical work of book preparation, I am grateful to Alan Schnur and Masanobu Sugimoto for their excellent advice and editing. I thank Ikuo Araki and Sakiko Maki for their persistent efforts in sorting out and recording the large amount of documentation necessary to prepare this book, and Sunaina Dalaya for her careful editing of the manuscript. I thank Sanjoy Bhattacharya for his advice and guidance on the publication of this book.

Lastly, I thank Mainichi Press, Nova Science Publishers and a few medical journals (as credited in the corresponding pages of the book) for permission to use their published materials. A very special thanks to the World Health Organization for permission to use their substantial data in the form of figures and tables and their meeting documentary materials.

Abbreviations

BWC	Biological Weapons Convention
CDC	Centers for Disease Control and Prevention
DPT	Diptheria, Pertussis and Tetanus (combined vaccine)
FDA	Flood and Drug Administration
GOARN	Global Outbreak Alert and Response Agency
JICA	Japan International Cooperation Agency
NIPH	National Institute of Public Health
OPV	Oral Polio Vaccine
UNDRO	United Nations Disaster Relief Organization
SEARO	South-East Asia Regional Office
WHA	World Health Assembly
WHO	World Health Organization

1

Smallpox in a Tropical Rain Forest in West Africa

I was walking in the tropical rain forest in Liberia, West Africa, in the winter of 1963. I was with eight Liberian smallpox control team members, together with ten Liberian porters who were carrying our equipment and luggage. We entered small hamlets every two to three hours during our walk. The three to five huts of the villages were made of thatch and poles, made from small tree branches. The villagers were glad to see us newcomers, and served us a few fruits to quench our thirst. We had started early in the morning, at six o'clock, but it was getting late, already dusk.

From time to time, there were heavy rain showers, turning the narrow forest path into a stream. This deep forest consisted of trees, 20–30 metres high, and ground covered by low bushes. We did not see any animals, but my Liberian colleagues said that they were there; we simply did not recognise them.

In 1962, I had come to Liberia as a World Health Organization (WHO) medical officer. It was my first experience in Africa. My job was to help the Liberian government implement a smallpox vaccination project as part of the global smallpox eradication programme. As part of the job, I had to investigate the number of smallpox cases and the manner in which the smallpox vaccination programme was being implemented.

The forest where I was walking was within Grand Bassa county. It was only 70 kilometres away from the Liberian capital, Monrovia. An officer of the Ministry of Health, Monrovia, told me that there were several smallpox cases there. Thus we entered the forest, figuring that with a 50 kilometre walk we would reach the spot where the smallpox cases were reported.

Suddenly the forest ended and there was an open area with a village in front of us. There were about twenty huts in the village, and we were welcomed by the smiling village chief. Lamps were shining, as it was already dark. I stayed at the village chief's house, and the team members at other houses or huts. I laid myself on the bed and put out the lamp. I could hear something moving in the ceiling. In addition, there was some local music, making *toko, toko* sounds in the distance. I fell asleep quickly due to fatigue. I did not know how long I slept, but suddenly I was awakened by one of my colleagues screaming: "Dr, Dr, Black ants! Black ants coming. Careful! Are your ears alright?" They were carrying torches and used them to clear the ants from the walls and floor.

Next morning we began our investigation with sleepy eyes. The smallpox surveillance methodology called for us to search for rash and fever patients in every hamlet within a 5 kilometre radius from this village. Some time before noon, I entered a hamlet and found a child with fresh pock marks. "Do you have other children with marks like these?" I asked. While I was asking, many other villagers appeared, and when they approached me, I found that almost half of them had similar marks on their faces. The villagers said, "There is a camp in the next valley with all the patients with rash and fever like this one!" With my team I went down the valley that everybody had pointed out with their fingers.

There I found about twenty smallpox patients suffering from fever and rash. A few villagers were helping them. A baby, whose whole body was covered by pustules, was being breastfed by the mother, who was at the crusting stage of smallpox. A young boy, also at the crusting stage, was helping to fill water into containers, standing close to the mother.

I spoke with them one by one through my Liberian interpreter and this is what they had to say:

> It is good here because we have water.
> Food can be brought here from the nearby hamlet.
> Every four or five years this disease comes to us.
> Vaccination? What is it? We never heard of this.
> You are the first doctor who has come to us from overseas.

The next three days were busy. We discovered 230 smallpox cases, prepared their case histories and epidemiological records, and provided simple drugs such as vitamins and anti-malaria tablets. Then we returned to Monrovia. At the time, the population in Liberia was about 1.5 million, with 90 per cent living in the bush without a hospital or health centre. Most people might never see a trained doctor or nurse in their entire lives. Smallpox was quietly attacking people, as I had seen with my Liberian colleagues, without the outside world aware of it.

In 1964, I completed my work in Liberia and other states in West Africa, and was re-assigned to work at the WHO headquarters in Geneva, Switzerland. In retrospect, my two years in Africa seemed to have passed in a moment, very rapidly; nevertheless, it was an extremely valuable experience for me. At the WHO headquarters, I was responsible for looking at and thinking of smallpox eradication from a global viewpoint. But whenever the situation became critical, my memories of Africa returned.

What I describe here occurred in 1964, almost half a century ago, but in 1958, five years earlier, WHO had already initiated a smallpox eradication programme throughout the world. However, the programme progressed in substantial difficulty with just one medical officer posted at the WHO headquarters in the Virological Diseases Unit covering the entire global programme, and supported by only a few additional staff at country level. During the first year of my Geneva assignment, I was instructed to prepare a draft strategic plan for an intensified smallpox eradication programme. I visited several countries, such as Mali, Nigeria, Afghanistan and Burma, where the smallpox eradication work was supposed to be ongoing. Except for Burma, I was convinced that a situation similar to Liberia was not uncommon in many developing areas. I found smallpox cases in one of the countries and said to the health minister, "I saw several cases of smallpox in the capital, why don't you report them?" The minister replied, "You are an officer of WHO. You should remember that I can decide how many cases we have. If I say no cases, it means there are really no cases". In one country, when I wanted to see the vaccination work done, the programme health officer responsible did not know where the vaccination teams were working!

These, and other findings during my visits, made it clear that if smallpox eradication was to succeed, WHO needed to do something on a war footing with sufficient funding.

2

Spring 1966: *WHO Executive Board Debates*

In Geneva, the lake reflects the silhouette of a large whitish building. This is the world famous *Palais des Nations*, or Palace of Nations, which was built after the First World War for the promotion of world peace. At the time of the meeting of the World Health Organization Executive Board (EB) in 1966, the WHO headquarter offices were situated in this building; in 1967, the headquarters were moved to a building on Avenue Appia where it remains to this day.

In January 1966, the EB met at the Palais des Nations to discuss the 1967 fiscal year regular WHO budget, which included, as the priority budget item, intensified global smallpox eradication. Prior to the budget proposal, the smallpox eradication programme was funded exclusively by donations and not through the regular budget, which is based on assessed payments from all WHO member states.

Marcolino Candau, the then WHO Director-General, informed the EB that,

> Smallpox eradication has now reached a turning point. Eight years have passed since the inception of the program in 1958, but the disease is still endemic in South America, sub-Saharan Africa and South East Asia. Progress has been very slow. Without increased efforts, it is not conceivable that we can achieve the target within a reasonable time schedule.
>
> Man is the only natural reservoir of smallpox. It is already well established that vaccination can interrupt person to person transmission. We know that smallpox disappeared in some geographical regions and continents through vaccination. Eradication is feasible. Then why do we still have endemic smallpox in the areas mentioned above?

> Because the public health systems in these countries are still at a developing stage, they have no effective census, no sensitive surveillance and no smallpox vaccine production! People are not aware of health issues, hence it is very difficult to achieve vaccination coverage high enough to stop the spread of the disease. No epidemiological studies have been conducted there. Sufficient resources are not available. Eight years have already elapsed now after smallpox eradication was initiated, relying mainly on the limited resources of the poorest nations.
>
> It is absolutely necessary to provide resources from outside if the program is to succeed. Therefore, WHO has now prepared a plan for an intensified 10-year program for the global eradication of smallpox, and we propose to the EB that US $2.5 million be allocated from regular budget every year to accomplish this plan.

This plan was prepared by me, with assistance from Donald A. Henderson, who had come to Geneva as a WHO consultant to assist in the plan preparation and supported the programme for smallpox eradication and measles control in western and central Africa. Karel Raska, Director of the WHO Division of Communicable Diseases, also supported the plan. Preparation of the budget was simple: the costing was based on the number of persons requiring vaccination, the number of vaccinators, the number of transport vehicles and cost of the required amount of vaccine. We also estimated the costs pertaining to external support needed for countries to cover the target population in three years.

Candau's proposal provoked extensive discussion among the EB members. At the time, the WHO annual budget was about US $45–50 million. An additional smallpox eradication programme budget of US $2.5 million would mean a 5 per cent increase. Furthermore, the 1967 WHO budget already contained a 6 per cent increase to cover inflation and the increased costs of things like travel, meetings and salaries. Together with the 5 per cent increase for smallpox eradication the total would thus increase to 11 per cent. EB members questioned whether such a huge increment in the regular budget was justified. Was eradication of a disease like smallpox really required?

An EB member expressed some of these feelings clearly during discussions:

> The problem of developing nations is not only smallpox but also many diseases such as encephalitis, diarrhea, malnutrition, water supply, lack of medical interventions and, above all, lack of basic health services. WHO regular budget is extremely limited. Why should we spend such a significant percentage of the total budget for a single disease like smallpox?

Another EB member expressed reservations about the feasibility of achieving the eradication goal: "In Asia and Africa people live and die without seeing a doctor. Nomads roam in the remote desert with camels and goats. How is it possible to vaccinate such people? How can you find smallpox cases in such areas?"

Such scepticism was also heavily influenced by delays in achieving malaria eradication. At the time, the WHO malaria eradication programme, which started in 1955, three years before the commencement of smallpox eradication, was failing. Technically, malaria eradication efforts suffered from mosquito resistance to DDT insecticide, as well as from surveillance difficulties due to a large number of sub-clinical infections. But the fundamental problem of the malaria programme was that it required a great deal of funds to implement the strategy, funds which were often not available in malaria endemic countries. For example, in India and Pakistan, at the height of the programme, more than 30 per cent of these two countries' health budgets were being spent on malaria eradication. Eventually, in the mid-1970s, the programme's problems led the WHO to re-orient the malaria eradication programme to malaria control, thus abandoning the eradication goal.

An European EB member proposed a compromise plan:

> I understand what the DG is aiming at. But this budgetary increment to promote measures against a single disease is excessive, given that it may lead to reduced funding for other important health programs. Let us start the 10-year program slowly. I would propose to start with US $1 million instead of US $2.5 million.

A few members seemed to support this proposal, but the Director-General argued strongly for his proposal.

> The World Health Assembly resolved that WHO implement smallpox eradication. The WHO secretariat in consultation with global experts

> studied the current situation for a few years and has now prepared this plan. This program will not succeed without outside assistance. The requested amount of US $2.5 million represents only one third of the total required budget for smallpox eradication. The remainder will be provided by the countries themselves. Also, this WHO budget for smallpox eradication should be from regular budget, because special budgets are at the mercy of donors and are not reliable and stable. For this eradication program, we need stable funding which permits continuous efforts every year over the next ten years. Without adequate and stable funding I don't believe that I can take responsibility to succeed in the eradication of smallpox as required by the WHA resolution.

Finally, a member from an East European nation intervened saying,

> I don't think that US $2.5 million is an enormous amount. Think that the USA spends US $140 million for its smallpox program including vaccination, surveillance, control and treatment of complications caused by smallpox vaccination. Great Britain spent US $2 million to control an imported smallpox outbreak recently. I believe that the amount of money for smallpox control that the industrialised nations spend every year globally is enormous. This is only because there is the risk of smallpox importations from smallpox endemic nations. If the eradication program succeeds and diminishes the risk, vaccination could be discontinued and no more expenditures would be required to control imported smallpox. This would lead to enormous savings and the cost of US $2.5 million would be minimal. Let us unify to fight smallpox. We can succeed if we collect all available technology and wisdom, overcome the differences of nations, races and politics. I shall support this proposal for a 10-year program to eradicate smallpox world wide.

The EB members from Africa, Asia and South America supported this statement. Finally, the EB voted and, by the margin of only two votes, decided to support the budget proposal to establish the programme. Thus, the May 1966 EB meeting resulted in the World Health Assembly (WHA) meeting in May of the same year, in which the WHA endorsed the EB decision, and passed a resolution on global smallpox eradication as follows: (i) That the WHO regular budget includes $2.5 million every year to be used for the ten-year programme of smallpox eradication starting in 1967; and

(ii) the WHO member states are urgently requested to promote the intensified programme making all necessary preparations.

Before detailing the actual programme implementation, it would be useful to review the characteristics of smallpox as a great and severe scourge, in terms of the clinical picture, epidemiology and control measures, including vaccination (as done in chapter 3). This is most appropriate given that only very few people living today have ever seen a case of smallpox. As was promised at the end of the smallpox eradication programme, this disease is now relegated to history books.

3

Smallpox: The Target Disease for Eradication

Smallpox is caused by the smallpox (variola) virus belonging to the Pox virus group (see figure 3.1). The only way the virus survives in nature is by being transmitted from person to person. Technically, human beings are the only natural reservoir of the smallpox virus. The virus cannot survive for long periods outside a human body, in the outside environment. Hence, if the virus is removed from all human beings, it would mean the end of the disease and the extinction of the smallpox virus.

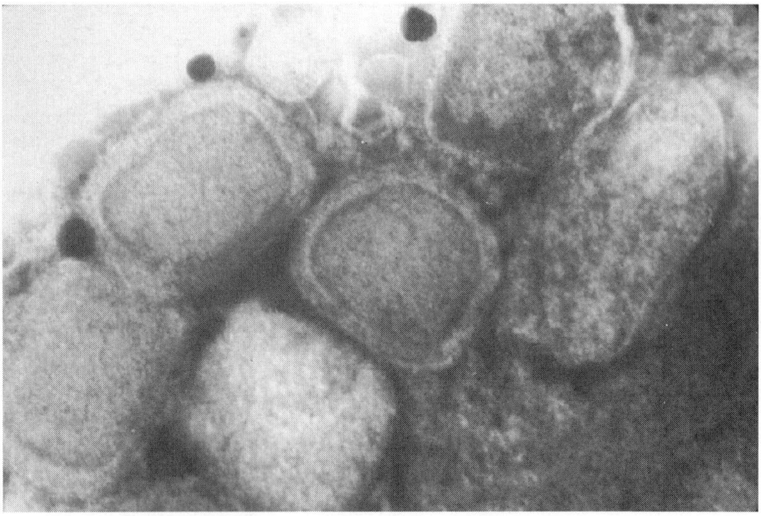

FIGURE 3.1 Variola minor seen using electron microscopy

Note: Specimen taken from the world's last case.
Source: World Health Organization.

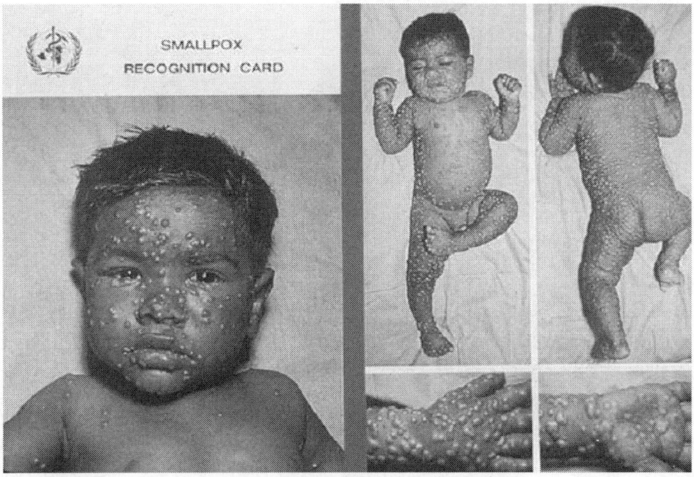

FIGURE 3.2 Smallpox recognition card used for surveillance

Source: World Health Organization.

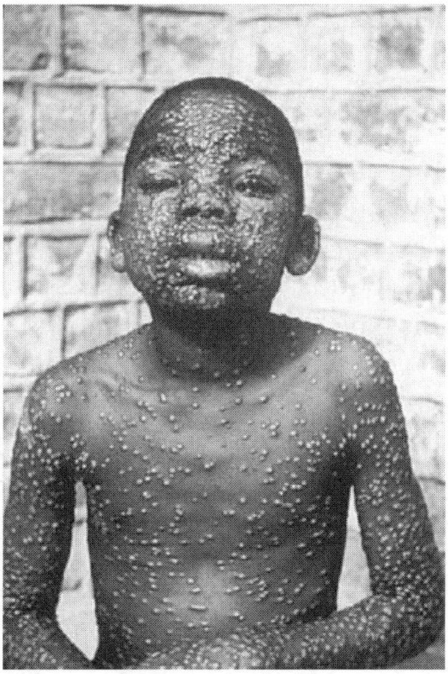

FIGURE 3.3 Typical case of smallpox, Zaire

Source: World Health Organization.

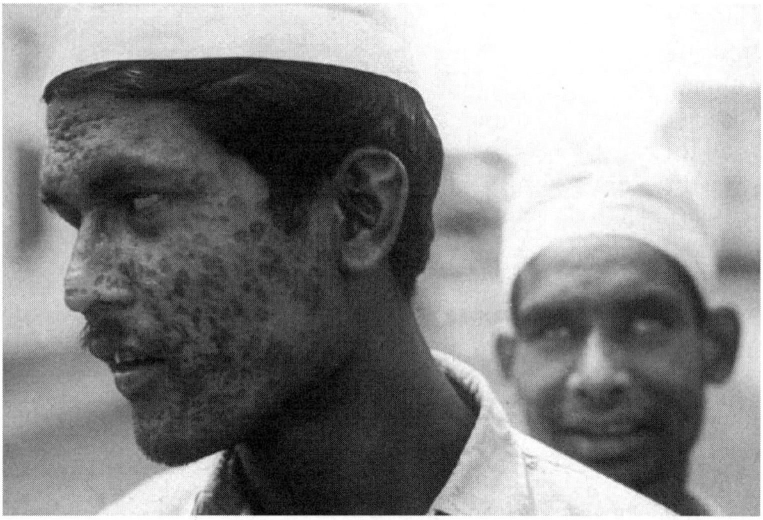

FIGURE 3.4 Typical pockmarks and blindness following smallpox, Bangladesh

Source: World Health Organization.

The smallpox virus normally infects humans through the respiratory route. After a twelve-day incubation period from the time of infection, the virus causes headaches, fever and muscular pain for three to four days, before causing a rash on the skin. The skin eruptions start first as an erythema, and then become papules, vesicles and pustules, taking about a week to progress to the pustule stage. The smallpox rash is typically distributed mostly on the extremities and face, and less on the trunk of the body (see figures 3.1 and 3.2). The different stages of the rash proceed evenly from erythema to pustule, with the many eruptions normally all at the same stage. At the last stage, the eruptions form crusts, and desquamations take place over the two weeks after pustule formation.

During this process, 20 to 30 per cent of smallpox patients die. If they survive, many are left with facial scarring, with pockmarks for the rest of their lives. In some cases, if the skin eruptions have affected the eyes, there is blindness (see figure 3.4). Thus, as can be imagined, the smallpox disease was greatly feared by people, some of whom worshipped a smallpox goddess or god to help them escape from the disease. The origin of the smallpox virus and disease is estimated to date back 6,000 years. One theory has the smallpox virus as originating in central Africa, from where it eventually spread to all the continents.[1]

In the late eighteenth century, Edward Jenner, an English country physician, developed a vaccine against smallpox. He noted that cowpox—a rash disease with some similarities to a mild form of smallpox—seemed to protect milkmaids, and thus might provide protection against smallpox. He famously tested his theory by inoculating a boy with a small amount of specimen taken from the lesion of a hand of young woman who had been accidentally infected by a cow, and showing that the inoculated boy was not infected with smallpox after inoculation of smallpox material. This idea and test began the process which eventually led to the development of the smallpox vaccine and its mass production. Use of the new vaccine spread rapidly and widely in Europe. It affected life expectancy, with life expectancy increasing between the eighteenth and nineteenth centuries from about twenty-five to forty years in France, and from about thirty-five to forty-five years in Sweden. Donald Hopkins, staff member of the US-based Centers for Disease Control and Prevention (CDC), who worked in the smallpox eradication programme, has written a book entitled *Princes and Peasants,* describing how smallpox affected human history by causing the deaths or illness of political leaders and members of royal families, and of peasants and lay people alike. For example, American president Abraham Lincoln, Mary II of England and Louis XV of France all suffered from smallpox, with the last two dying of the disease.[2]

The introduction of the smallpox vaccine greatly altered the aforementioned situation. Later, improvements were made in the production process of the vaccine, and it was made heat stable using techniques developed by Leslie Collier of the United Kingdom,

[1] Norman Howard-Jones, "Thousand-year Scourge", *World Health*, February–March 1975, 4–11.

[2] Donald R. Hopkins, *Princes and Peasants: Smallpox in History* (Chicago: University of Chicago Press, 1983).

who invented lyophilisation or freeze drying technology. The heat stable vaccine proved to be indispensable for smallpox eradication in tropical areas where refrigerators were not readily available, or if available, were often not in working condition.

The epidemiology of smallpox was better understood before the intensified phase of the programme was initiated. A. Ramachandra Rao (Madras, India), discovered that the transmission of smallpox requires close contact, and that the infection rate when exposed to a patient may not be high, resulting in a secondary case in only about 40 per cent of family contacts. This was an important finding. The US-West Africa bilateral programme had also shown that smallpox did not spread rapidly and needed close contact for transmission.[3] Also, during the programme, there was a general understanding that a high population density tended to sustain the continuous transmission of smallpox. I published an article on this with John Wickett and Frank Fenner in 1986.[4] These findings were important epidemiological observations and affected the development of the surveillance and containment strategy of the smallpox programme. Hence, they are noted here specifically.

Now, having described the essential features of smallpox as the target disease for global eradication, let us return to the initial phase of the intensified programme, as determined by the 1966 WHA.

[3] R. H. Henderson and M. Yekpe, "Smallpox Transmission in Southern Dahomey: A Study of a Village Outbreak", *American Journal of Epidemiology* 90, no. 5, 1969, 423–28.

[4] I. Arita, J. Wickett and F. Fenner, "Impact of Population Density on Immunization Programmes", *Journal of Hygiene* 96, 1986, 459–66.

4

Initial Phase of Launching the Intensified Smallpox Eradication Programme

In 1967, following the WHA resolution, the WHO initiated the intensified global programme of smallpox eradication. The strategy was modified as the programme proceeded, but here we describe the overall plans of the initial strategies followed.

1. In 1967, there were thirty-three countries where smallpox was endemic (smallpox had always been present and there was ongoing transmission). In these countries, the entire population needed to be vaccinated, up to at least 80 per cent coverage within three years (see figure 4.1). It was expected that raising immunisation coverage levels to 80 per cent or above would reduce the number of cases sufficiently so that intensive local vaccination could be organised to stop transmission.
2. It was decided that the smallpox vaccine used should meet WHO standards. To assure that the vaccine quality was good in terms of potency, two WHO collaborating laboratories were established to test the stability and safety of the vaccine lots for programme use. It was also decided that the local vaccine production system should be promoted.
3. It was decided that smallpox surveillance should be strengthened.
4. Finally, research was to be encouraged, especially on the reservoir of the smallpox virus.

To implement these strategies, WHO set up a smallpox eradication unit at its headquarters in Geneva, with four medical officers: D. A. Henderson (USA), S. Falkland (UK), N. Gorgij Nikolaevsky (USSR) and myself (Japan). An additional staff of six supported us, and included administrative officers and secretaries.

Map 4.1 Smallpox endemic countries and those with importations, 1967

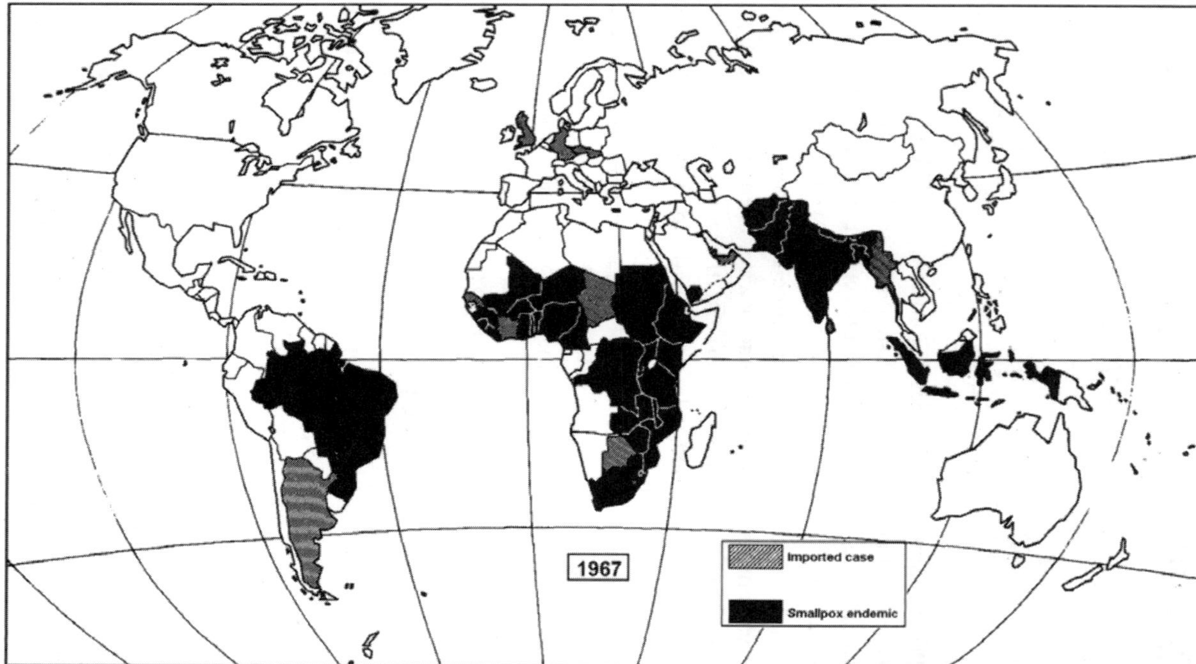

Source: World Health Organization.

D. A. Henderson and I worked together over the next ten years, but the other two original medical officers left WHO within a few years. Henderson was the first chief of the Smallpox Eradication Unit, having built a strong programme with his excellent technical capability and leadership. He left Geneva for Baltimore in February 1977 to become dean of the Johns Hopkins University School of Hygiene and Public Health. I replaced him as chief of the unit for the final phase of the programme; this included the final battle against the virus in the Horn of Africa (where the last naturally occurring smallpox case was discovered in Somalia in October 1977), and the process of certifying smallpox eradication that culminated with certification by the WHA in May 1980 of the global interruption of smallpox transmission. During the period, Henderson and I were able to sustain a close personal contact despite the long distance between Geneva and Baltimore.

At the WHO regional office level, medical officers were appointed as Regional Advisers in the three smallpox endemic regions of Africa, South-East Asia and the Eastern Mediterranean. At the country level, one WHO medical officer was appointed in almost all smallpox endemic countries. If the country had a large population, as in the case of India and Brazil, more than one medical officer was assigned. So, although it may have looked like the global smallpox programme had a strong system, it was not so. By comparison, at the time, the failing malaria eradication programme had a staff of 534, with an annual budget of US $14 million. Our smallpox eradication programme had no more than forty to fifty personnel with an annual budget of US $2.5 million. Needless to say, at the country level, national governments and ministries of health were expected to use their own budgets to conduct smallpox eradication activities. However, as seen in the Liberian programme, it was not uncommon that in endemic countries national teams had neither the transport nor travelling expenses to respond to smallpox outbreaks.

In such a scenario, there were huge obstacles to overcome in order to treat the total smallpox affected population of two billion, with an estimated smallpox incidence of twenty million cases per year throughout the world. I recall how a few high-ranking WHO officials did not think smallpox eradication was feasible. For example, during the WHO Executive Board (EB) session in spring 1966, when the smallpox budget was approved, an Assistant Director-General of WHO commented to me, "As you know, soldiers march to the battlefield knowing that they will be defeated; likewise WHO now will march for smallpox eradication knowing that we will fail." I would like to point out that the gentleman in question was a competent health officer with good management skills.

I once heard a rumour that the then Director-General, Marcolino Candau, himself did not believe in the feasibility of smallpox eradication, based on the situation in the Amazon river basin. In remote areas, health officials did not know where the natives lived and died, or even how many there were. Thus, in such a situation would it be possible to vaccinate them all? In this case, eradication would be impossible. Perhaps this was Marcolino Candau's personal insight, but I believe the way he defended the smallpox budget during the 1966 EB session indicated his superb ability and determination as the head of WHO to follow the WHA's initial recommendation to eradicate the disease. In hindsight, with the experience gained during the programme, we now know that the smallpox virus cannot easily survive in the conditions found in the Amazon. Without a more dense population and close contact between people, the virus dies out naturally.

The eradication programme also presented difficulties vis-à-vis the vaccination techniques available. While in Liberia, I studied the efficacy of vaccination using one model of the jet injector (a machine that uses air pressure to push the vaccine into the skin). A missionary team from USA that was visiting Liberia had organised a smallpox vaccination session in Monrovia using the new vaccination method of the jet injector. I studied their jet injectors with my Liberian colleagues by revaccinating the vaccinees again using the usual vaccination method of scarification. The revaccination produced a take rate of 40 per cent, suggesting that the vaccination done using the jet injector had poor efficacy. The leader of the missionary team was angry at my finding, and wrote to the WHO Director-General requesting my dismissal for criticising his work. Candau immediately wrote back to me instructing me to ignore such criticism and to continue with my work. It was later that I learnt that the efficacy of this jet injector had also been questioned by some CDC experts in the US.

Despite the difficulties mentioned above, the morale of the smallpox team was high. Perhaps we were young and didn't believe in failure. Perhaps only those who were interested and motivated came to work for the programme. Whatever the reasons, we tried continuously to increase the efficacy of the programme as much as we could, and to encourage our colleagues at the national level to do the same. As I write this book, a few of my colleagues from the early stages of the programme cross my mind. It is unfortunate that space considerations make it possible to write about only a few of these outstanding people.

Nicole Grasset, medical virologist with the Pasteur Institute in Paris, came to work at the regional office for South-East Asia in New Delhi, India. She was dynamic, kind and straightforward. Once, one of her colleagues at the regional office commented, "If you can eradicate smallpox in India, I will eat the tyre of your car". We all knew that he would be made to eat the tyre of Nicole's car in May 1975.

William Foege, former leader of the USA bilateral assistance programme for smallpox eradication and measles control in West Africa, spent quite a bit of time helping the Indian smallpox eradication programme. Standing two metres tall, he had a special technique for getting sufficient legroom on the crowded Indian domestic flights. "Do you know how to sit in the plane?" he would ask. "I get into the cabin early, sit in a seat and cover my mouth with a paper sack. That way nobody comes to sit beside me." I believe he really did this because he liked to joke and was constantly innovating during his work. Subsequently, Foege went on to serve as Director of CDC, USA, with Donald Hopkins (another effective smallpox worker in the US bilateral programme in West Africa) as the Deputy Director.

Claudio Amaral, Director of the Brazilian national smallpox eradication programme, visited me at my office at the WHO headquarters in Geneva after the last case of smallpox in Brazil in 1971. He expressed his desire to work for WHO smallpox eradication. He acknowledged that he did not speak English well, but that his wife, Alba, would always be there to help him and so there would be no problem. After giving it much thought, I accepted. There were no problems at all. Claudio helped the programme very much, especially during the last battles in the Horn of Africa, always together with Alba.

Lastly, I comment retrospectively on the adequacy of the planned WHO budget for the intensified smallpox eradication programme established in 1966, and the actual expenditures up to the end of the programme in 1980 (see box 4.1).

Box 4.1 Initial estimates of the costs of the eradication effort

During the EB debate, a few members had commented that the regular smallpox budget was exceedingly expensive, taking 5 per cent of the total sum of WHO's annual regular budget. The following figures, showing the total national and international expenditures for smallpox eradication from 1967 to 1979, are taken from the WHO smallpox eradication certification committee report in 1979. In the end, the regular budget of smallpox eradication was "exceedingly" limited, and had to be supplemented by extra-budgetary funds or voluntary contributions from bilateral organisations. Three decades have passed. In retrospect, we now have the advantage of being able to review the level of funding that was made available and how much the national programmes, as well as the WHO support programme, had to struggle to be successful, despite the limited funding.

Given here is a total cost of the WHO intensified smallpox eradication programme from 1967 to 1979 (figures courtesy WHO).

WHO regular budget	$ 38 000 000
WHO voluntary fund for health promotion (donation)	$ 43 000 000
Bilateral aid	$ 32 000 000
Estimated national expenditure	$ 200 000 000
Total	$ 313 000 000

We originally estimated that with an annual allocation of US $2.5 million for ten years, the programme would need a total WHO regular budget of $25 million, for the ten years until eradication. With additional national budgets contributing the remaining two thirds of the total programme needs, $75 million would be the cost for the eradication effort. Certainly, at the inception of the programme in 1967, it would not have been easy to make an exact costing, but I must acknowledge that we grossly underestimated the cost, even when taking inflation into account.

The point is that despite such poor initial costing estimates, in addition to the logistical difficulties mentioned at the start of the global programme, it still succeeded. This was due in large part to the very harmonious joint efforts of the international community and programme staff, with a common final goal in mind. In other words, the programme did not suffer from the bureaucracy hampering the efficacy and effectiveness of the programme, perhaps due to the nature of the system, namely an ad hoc type of small group system. How and why did this happen? Hopefully, the next few chapters will answer these questions.

5

USA Bilateral Programme for Smallpox Eradication and Measles Control in West and Central Africa

In 1966, when the WHA resolved to initiate the intensified smallpox eradication programme, Karel Raska, Director of the Communicable Disease Division at the WHO headquarters, flew to Atlanta, USA, to discuss the programme with the staff of the CDC. Both WHO and the US health authorities agreed that the latter add smallpox eradication to its bilateral programme for measles control, which had already been scheduled in West and Central Africa. Thus, a US bilateral programme, with an annual budget of US$4 million, started to control measles and eradicate smallpox in nineteen African countries, with a combined population of 120 million, from Senegal in the west to Cameroon in Central Africa. This budget was much larger than that of the WHO global budget of US $2.5 million. The headquarters for the programme was set up in Lagos, the then capital of Nigeria, with eight experts from the US. In each of the nineteen countries, national offices were established, with an additional staff of thirty-three experts from the US posted at the country level. In addition, eight more staff was posted at the CDC office in Atlanta, USA, to coordinate the programme. Necessary transportation and vaccines were also supplied by the US. The planning was jointly carried out with WHO, which also provided the budget for local expenses such as per-diem payments, petrol, vehicle maintenance, etc., which could not be provided from the USA-CDC budget.

During the West and Central Africa operation, substantial new technical findings and developments emerged that were to greatly benefit the global smallpox eradication programme (see box 5.1).

Box 5.1 Smallpox transmission and its critical study of epidemiology

R. Henderson, medical officer, CDC, USA, and M. Yekpe, medical officer, *Service National des Grandes Endemics,* Dahomey, investigated a smallpox outbreak in a village of about 300 people, living in sixty houses. The outbreak started on 25 May 1967 and continued for three months, with the last case occurring around 9 August. There were a total of twenty-eight cases of smallpox. However, interestingly enough, of the twenty-eight cases, twenty-one lived in six houses within a 10-yard radius. The first house, the one to contract smallpox first, had done so from another village. However, because the household members of these six houses had very close contact with each other, the rest too began to be infected with the virus. The remaining houses—seven, eight and nine—were at a distance from the cluster of infected houses. So, did they have any contact with the infected persons? The investigation revealed the following:

- In house seven, about 20 yards away from the first house, a boy often carried food to the infected houses.
- In house eight, about 50 yards away from the first house, a grand fetisheur lived, who had close contact with the smallpox patients during ritual practice as well as diagnosis.
- In house nine, about 80 yards away from the first house, lived a very close friend of the fetisheur, and he often visited the infected houses too.

Vaccination coverage in this village was about 10 per cent. The important point is that the outbreak was hidden until mid-August. This means that the outbreak subsided before intervention began and before the vaccinations became effective. Three lessons emerge from this investigation: first, smallpox infection requires close contact; second, it spreads slowly; third, the transmission could naturally stop if supply of susceptibles with close contact is not sustained.

These simple but clear lessons contributed to the development of the surveillance and containment theory; the most important discovery for the success of the smallpox eradication programme, from my personal viewpoint, and comparable to the vaccine discovery by Edward Jenner in the late eighteenth century.

Source: Henderson and Yekpe, "Smallpox Transmission on Southern Dahomey".

The programme prepared and used operational manuals, full of practical, even if sometimes minor, guidance. For example, the manual suggested that "the driver who takes the team may sleep in the car while waiting for their return from field work". The manual was soon shared with all the WHO country programmes. The new jet injector was widely used for the first time, vaccinating 2,000 to 4,000 people a day. The jet injector also helped save smallpox vaccine (see figure 5.1), using only two thirds of the amount required for the traditional vaccination, and with a better take rate. As already mentioned in chapter 3 and box 5.1, M. Yekpe and R. H. Henderson clarified the pattern of smallpox spread in a village of Dahomey (currently Benin). When, one day, during the programme, the vaccine supply was short, one of the teams vaccinated only a portion of the inhabitants in the villages where cases were occurring. The result was amazing: the transmission ceased without mass vaccination of all the villages in the area. This was in fact the groundbreaking discovery that surveillance and containment could be the principal strategy to interrupt transmission instead of mass vaccination of the entire population.

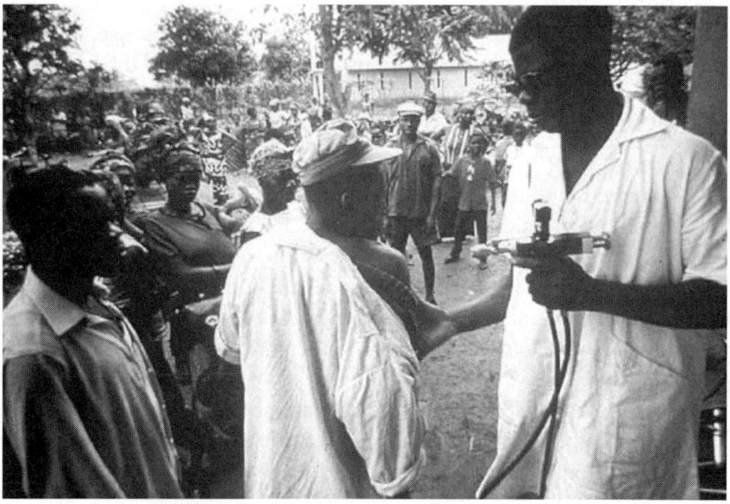

FIGURE 5.1 Jet injector in use, Central Africa

Source: World Health Organization

Another finding from the West Africa programme was that notification of smallpox cases was extremely poor. For example, in Nigeria it was estimated that less than 1 per cent of the actual number of cases occurring were reported. My experience in Liberia supported this estimate.

The CDC programme proceeded on schedule. In the first three years, 100 million vaccinations were carried out, with coverage reaching 80 per cent of the total population of the nineteen countries. Following the mass vaccination phase, after two years of operations using the surveillance and containment strategy, the last outbreak of sixty-six cases occurred in Nigeria in 1970. No cases were discovered in the nineteen countries of West and Central Africa in 1971, despites intensive surveillance in the programme areas.

William Foege later remarked (and this is from memory),

> The US spent $150 million annually for domestic smallpox related expenses. The West and Central Africa smallpox program, lasting from 1967 to 1970, cost a total of US $15 million. This corresponded to only 36 days of budget spent by the USA on smallpox. And this amount would need to be continued if the disease were not eradicated.

The smallpox eradication programme in West and Central Africa contributed in two major ways: (i) It eliminated a great source of misery for the people who were living in the poorest conditions over a large area, similar to conditions I had seen in Liberia (chapter 1); (ii) It proved that the WHA decision to eradicate smallpox was feasible even in diverse geographical areas with extreme poverty and the most limited health resources anywhere in the world.

To understand why Nigeria was the last country with smallpox at the time, I studied some old records. I found that Nigeria was the most densely populated country in West Africa, and that the surveillance and containment work was less effective here than in the other eighteen countries.[1] This was similar to findings from the programme in South Asia, where, in northern Pakistan, smallpox transmission was sustained in the densely populated Lahore area,

[1] Arita, Wickett and Fenner, "Impact of Population Density on Immunization Programmes".

while outbreaks in thinly populated rural surrounding areas died out naturally without containment vaccination.

Based on this experience of smallpox eradication, I note that the current polio eradication programme has been delayed, especially in Africa. Nigeria is the only remaining endemic country in Africa, and, as of December 2008, ten countries were still suffering importations from Nigeria, twenty years after the programme's inception. If a polio eradication programme had been organised in West and Central Africa at the start, as done by the CDC for smallpox eradication, the situation might have been very different for the currently delayed polio programme. In addition, many African countries began their polio eradication programmes only in the mid-1990s, around six or seven years after global polio eradication was started, in 1988. In hindsight, there is a lesson to be learnt. The global eradication of any disease requires strong global coordination efforts so that any delays to the programme can be avoided, if possible right from the beginning. In fact, this would be one of the most critical conditions for the successful interruption of the global transmission of any disease. I would like to add here that when the intensified smallpox eradication programme was started in 1967, special WHO teams immediately visited those nations that had not developed the intensified programme, and recommended that they start with the offer of new WHO transport and vaccines as needed.

At the time, in West Africa, the local people worshipped the smallpox god, Sopona. Priests would collect material from the lesions of smallpox patients, and inoculate children with it instead of the smallpox vaccine (variolation). When smallpox cases were disappearing in the region, the priests lacked the supply of the materials for variolation. In Dahomey (now Benin), when the last outbreak was being contained, many variolators rushed to meet the existing patient for collection of specimens (see figure 5.2).

In conclusion, of the nineteen countries where this programme was initiated in 1967, there were thirteen that reported smallpox cases; the highest reported number of smallpox cases was 4,700 and the lowest a single case. Please remember my Liberian experience: one case meant how many cases? In subsequent years, there was rapid reduction in the number of smallpox reporting countries: twelve in 1968, eight in 1969 and only one (Nigeria) in 1970. Eventually, zero smallpox cases were reported in all nineteen countries in West and Central Africa, despite the continuing surveillance activities in 1971. Thus, the smallpox eradication programme was successful in this region. How the programme progressed in the other regions and continents is examined in the following chapters.

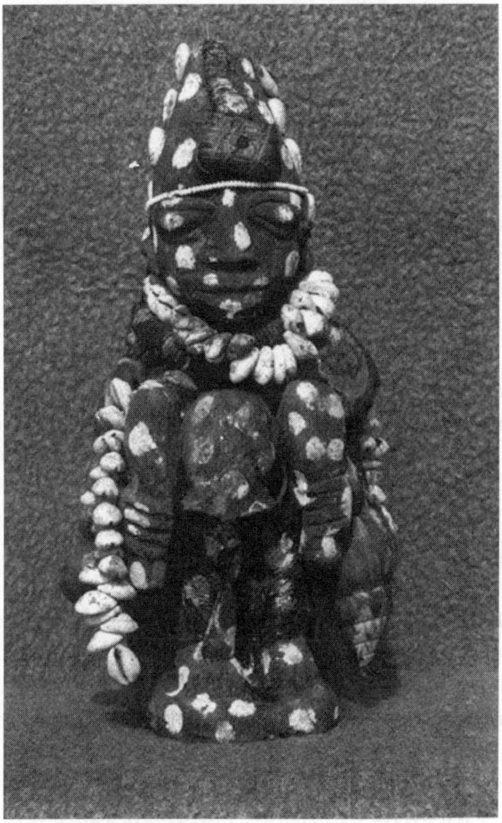

FIGURE 5.2 Sopona, smallpox god
Source: I. Arita, *Smallpox Eradication: Target Zero*.[2]

[2] Richard-Ernst Bader, "Sopono, Pocken und Pockengottkult der Yoruba". *Medizinhistorisches Journal* 21 (Stuttgart, New York: Gustav Fisher Verlag: 1986). Permission to reproduce by Olaf Meding.

6

Harbingers of the Intensified Programme

Originally, the smallpox eradication programme began in 1958, but, as mentioned before, the newly intensified programme only started in 1967, covering about thirty-three countries. Of course, at the time, these countries were extremely poor, with the least developed health resources as seen in Liberia (chapter 1). Further, there were other endemic diseases such as malaria and tuberculosis that had to be addressed, and were additional burdens to the extremely limited health budgets. Despite these difficulties, some of these remaining countries were already developing active and effective programmes during the early phase of the intensified programme. At the same time, this made it possible to use lessons from these countries to further strengthen the global smallpox eradication strategy. Brazil and Indonesia, two good examples, are described in this chapter.

Brazil, South America

The southern region of the Americas started an eradication programme of yellow fever in the 1920s and 1930s. Unfortunately, the effort failed because it was discovered that the yellow fever virus could be preserved in non-human primates of the tropical rain forest in the Amazon Basin. However, armed with this experience, an eradication campaign per se was not new for many of the countries in the region, and by 1967 Brazil was the only country in the region with endemic smallpox. From 1967 to 1968, the Brazilians used jet injectors for mass campaigns (although a different model than the one used in Liberia), and in 1969 they started to employ the surveillance and containment strategy, following the lessons learnt in the West African programme.

In Brazil, the surveillance functioned well, with thousands of reporting units distributed throughout the country. Claudio Amaral was an excellent leader, and with outstanding fieldworkers like Ciro de Quadros, among others, guiding the operation it proceeded well. Many of the Brazil eradication programme veterans later served with the WHO global smallpox eradication effort, as well as with the polio and measles eradication efforts. The last case of smallpox was found in Brazil in 1971. Interestingly enough, it occurred in Rio de Janeiro, a big urban city, rather than in the remote Amazon basin that Marcolino Candau had worried about.

Indonesia, South Asia

At the start of the intensified programme, there were six smallpox endemic countries in South Asia: Afghanistan, Bangladesh, India, Indonesia, Nepal and Pakistan. Their health services were better compared to sub-Saharan Africa, but they usually stuck to the traditional eradication strategy, namely 100 per cent vaccination coverage with mass campaigns. However, health officials in Indonesia were more flexible and innovative. The Director-General for the Control and Prevention of Communicable Diseases, Julie Sulianti Saroso, said, "we started the nation-wide mass vaccination campaign, but think of the fact that only children remaining unvaccinated get smallpox. We are successfully vaccinating almost 80 per cent of the children. Why not to find the unvaccinated children and vaccinate them? In this way we can more rapidly eradicate smallpox". [1] When they started to search for unvaccinated children, they often found smallpox cases with a typical clinical picture. I visited Indonesia often, and listened with interest and pleasure to their discussions about the programme. They decided to stop the search for unvaccinated people. Instead, they changed the emphasis of their search and began to look for smallpox outbreaks, and then vaccinate the villagers and patient contacts in infected villages. Notably, they arrived independently at the same strategy as was developed by the programme in West and Central Africa.

Another problem for the programme in Indonesia, where an innovation was required, was of how to find smallpox effectively

[1] From author's memory.

and efficiently. Here again, Petrus Aswin Koswara, the national programme officer, suggested, "How about to make a photo of a smallpox case and show it to villagers? This will be much more effective than talking and asking them about smallpox cases". Finally, WHO agreed to use a photo, that was later termed the "smallpox recognition card". I myself often used this card when visiting in the field to investigate surveillance sensitivity.

The clinical picture of smallpox is distinctly clear, an advantage when carrying out surveillance for the disease. In fact, WHO produced several million copies of the smallpox recognition card during the global programme. In Indonesia, the last case was found in a village only 40 kilometres away from the capital, Jakarta, rather than in a remote area. This was a similar experience to the Brazilian programme, and again emphasised the importance of programme implementation in the areas of high population density to stop transmission of the disease.

Thus, in addition to the successful campaign in West and Central Africa, both the country programmes discussed here could be regarded as the forerunners of the smallpox eradication programme from a global viewpoint. Both countries had large populations and covered vast geographical areas; Indonesia had a large number of islands too! In both countries, the smallpox vaccine had been locally produced. The vaccine produced in Brazil never met WHO standards; nevertheless, it appears that this disadvantage was compensated for by the excellent performance of their surveillance and vaccination programme.[2] This was truly exceptional, and hence finds mention here.

[2] Fenner et al., *Smallpox and its Eradication*.

7

Was the Smallpox Vaccine Good Enough to Start the Programme?

Were we certain that the smallpox vaccine being used in the programme, the principal tool for eradication, was of good quality? For if the vaccine being used was not good, all efforts would fail.

It was true that, at the time, the available smallpox vaccine was effective enough to allow many industrialised countries to interrupt smallpox transmission with it. North America, Europe, Japan and a few developing regions and countries were free of endemic smallpox, although they continued to suffer frequent importations. In these geographical regions, the vaccine products had been improved year by year too. First, the vaccine strain widely used in the vaccine was no longer made from the cowpox virus used in Edward Jenner's time (chapter 3). The vaccinia virus, belonging to the same pox virus family, was used; and there were increasingly more strains being used in production systems, mainly in industrialised countries. Parenthetically, it is interesting to note that since the period of Louis Pasteur and Robert Koch in the nineteenth century, discussions have continued over the origin of the vaccinia virus, and whether it is the current vaccine seed virus for the production of the smallpox vaccine. Derrick Baxby, a retired senior lecturer in medical microbiology at Liverpool University, UK, observed that " . . . increasingly sophisticated studies of the DNA of the viruses now show that cowpox, smallpox and vaccinia virus are independent species. . . . The enigma posed by the missing horsepox which, as grease [horsepox], played an important role in Jenner's thoughts and was widely used in some nineteenth century vaccines". Thus, "[the] vaccinia virus probably represents the laboratory survival of the otherwise extinct horsepoxs virus" he analysed and concluded.[1]

The search for better vaccine strains was driven by the concern that the smallpox vaccine caused severe reactions in some of the vaccinees—such as post-vaccinal encephalitis, progressive vaccinia and eczema vaccinatum—although this was infrequent. The frequency of such complications varied with different strains of the vaccinia virus; but the American experience found that, on average, post-vaccinal encephalitis occurred in ten vaccinees per million primary vaccinations, progressive vaccinia in four vaccinees per million, and eczema vaccinatum in forty-one vaccinees per million.[2] The first two reactions often caused severe complications, including death. In addition there were other reactions, often requiring hospitalisation, including generalised vaccinia or accidental infection by exposure to persons who had been vaccinated, which were less severe, but nonetheless occurred in a few hundred vaccinees or their contacts per year. The complications were much less for re-vaccinations. The point was that despite these complications, countries free of endemic smallpox had to implement regular and uniform vaccination programmes to immunise their population and protect them against a smallpox importation. One of the major reasons why these countries strongly supported the smallpox eradication effort was because they assumed that vaccination could be discontinued after the eradication.

In 1967, D. A. Henderson and I had detailed discussions on the vaccine required for the global programme while reviewing the vaccine supply record available at our office. The following is from one such conversation:

> We need at least 300 million doses of vaccine of good quality annually, but we do not know the true quality of the vaccine currently available, including some of that which will be donated to WHO. How can we be

[1] Derrick Baxby, *Smallpox Vaccine: Ahead of its Time* (Barkley, UK: The Jenner Museum, 2001).

[2] J. M. Lane, F. L. Ruben, J. M. Neff and J. D. Millar, "Complications of Smallpox Vaccination, 1968. National Surveillance in the United States". *New England Journal of Medicine* 281, no. 22, 1969, 1201–8.

assured that there are sufficient donations and supply of good quality vaccine?

We agreed that there were many unanswered questions concerning smallpox vaccine supply. The WHO needed to know (a) how much vaccine was being produced throughout the world, (b) how 300 million doses of vaccine yearly could be made available to the intensified smallpox eradication effort, and (c) what would be the quality of the vaccine. Accordingly, WHO sent a carefully prepared letter to the heads of the health services in each country. Perhaps, readers will consider this action on the part of WHO as ordinary; however, at the time, the letter caused adverse reactions from some member states, who wondered why the WHO doubted their vaccine quality. For example, one country said, "Don't you trust our good control of the quality of smallpox vaccines?" As a result, WHO had to patiently and carefully explain the rationale behind the letter to many delegations from the member states.

In the end, the information collected did show some surprising findings. There were fifty-nine production laboratories of freeze-dried smallpox vaccine in twenty-eight countries. Of the production lots tested by the WHO collaborating centres for smallpox vaccine, only 30 per cent met WHO standards. Some of the lots failed the potency testing, while some the heat stability test, and others were found to be contaminated (an excessive bacterial count). We suspected that since the test sample specimens sent by individual laboratories were probably the best ones, the real situation was far worse. We suspected that the actual percentage of lots that met WHO standards could be much lower, less than 10 per cent! This raised the question of how WHO could get enough vaccine of good quality to meet the needs of the intensified programme. Further, based on the cost of US $0.01 per dose, 300 million dose vaccines would cost US $3 million, against the total annual programme budget of US $2.5 million. Clearly, even if the WHO needed to buy the vaccine, it would be unable to do so since the cost would exceed the allocated budget for personnel, transport and travel. The programme therefore included, in the original plan, to acquire the vaccine free of cost through donations. As mentioned, there were huge problems with the quality and supply of the vaccine in the first two years of the intensified programme.What was the solution to these two problems?

First, several countries, including USA, Canada, USSR, the Netherlands and UK, agreed to donate the vaccine (as per WHO standards) immediately as a contingency action in order to help the programme work get started. However, for the ten-year programme, it was necessary to develop a sustainable plan for sufficient vaccine supply of assured quality. The WHO urgently set up a special expert group to prepare a simple manual for the production of the smallpox vaccine and assay procedures. I participated in their work and was impressed with the fact that the experts worked hard to develop a simple and user-friendly manual by applying the know-how from their own production technology. This seemed unusual from a market-oriented point of view. The manuals were distributed to all the production laboratories. The experts advising WHO came from the laboratories in Europe and North America, including Connaught Medical Research Laboratory, Canada; National Institute of Public Health (NIPH), the Netherlands; Wyeth Laboratories, USA; Lister Institute, UK; and the Research Institute of Viral Preparations, USSR.

The first two of the aforementioned laboratories were designated as WHO Collaborating Reference Laboratories for Smallpox Vaccine. Connaught was to cover the American region, and the NIPH, the Netherlands the rest of the world. During the entire period of the intensified programme, these institutes devoted staff time and resources towards providing guidance on vaccine production and testing, as well as for testing the vaccine samples received from production facilities around the world. [3]

As shown in table 7.1, the vaccine quality started to improve in the third year of the programme. It is important to note that all the vaccine lots donated to the WHO for use in the intensified programme were tested by the WHO Collaborating Laboratories, and on failing the tests were not used for the programme. Consequently,

[3] I. Arita, "The Control of Vaccine Quality in the Smallpox Eradication Programme", in *Symposia Series in Immuno-biological Standardization* 19, 1972, 78–87, International Symposium on Smallpox Vaccine, Bilthoven, The Netherlands, 11–13 October 1972 (Basel: Karger 1973).

TABLE 7.1 WHO testing of smallpox vaccine batches, 1967–80

Year	*Number of producers*	*Number of batches submitted*	*Number satisfactory (%)*	*Number unsatisfactory (%)*	*Unsatisfactory*		
					Initial potency	*Heat stability*	*Bacterial count*
1967	20	74	27 (36)	47 (64)	32	12	8
1968	23	136	74 (54)	62 (46)	26	36	5
1969	30	164	128 (78)	36 (22)	23	12	5
1970	27	380	312 (82)	68 (18)	27	35	13
1971	32	206	154 (75)	52 (25)	31	23	5
1972	27	311	241 (77)	70 (23)	32	39	1
1973	30	392	367 (94)	25 (6)	5	20	0
1974	28	231	199 (86)	32 (14)	11	20	1
1975	21	167	139 (83)	28 (17)	15	10	6
1976	16	213	203 (95)	10 (5)	2	7	3
1977	11	114	101 (89)	13 (11)	1	12	1
1978	9	59	57 (97)	2 (3)	0	2	0
1979	10	85	82 (96)	3 (4)	3	1	0
1980	5	46	46 (100)	0 (–)	0	0	0
Total	—	2,578	2,130 (82.6)	448 (17.4)	208	229	48

Source: Fenner et al., *Smallpox and its Eradication*.

better quality control improved the quality of the vaccine used in the programme, but increased the difficulty of having sufficient vaccine supplies to meet demand. However, here we were helped by a few developing countries that had started to locally produce good quality vaccine in their own production facilities. During the late phase of the programme, in the 1970s, the following countries were producing the smallpox vaccine for their own use: Colombia, Brazil, India, Indonesia, Bangladesh and Kenya (see figure 7.1).

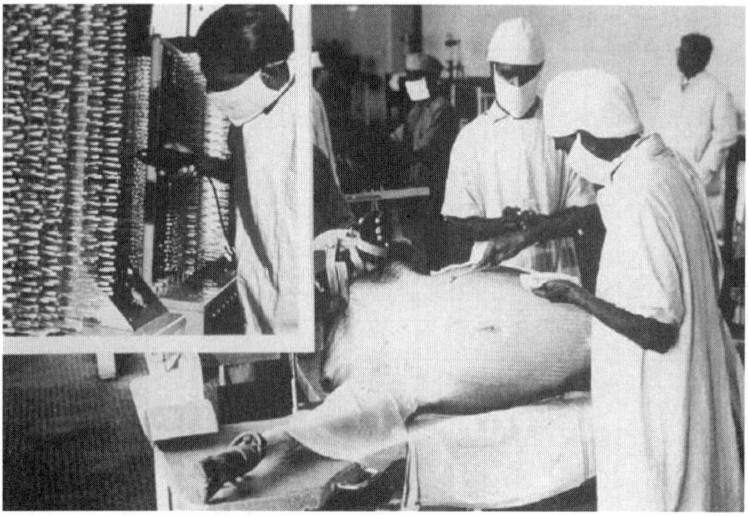

FIGURE 7.1 Smallpox vaccine production in India, 1970s

Source: World Health Organization.

Lastly, the smallpox vaccine had an added operational advantage. The vaccine could sustain its potency for four weeks at 40° C (as discussed in chapter 3). It was thus important to ensure that the heat stability of the vaccine was adequate, and WHO made some innovations to speed up the laboratory testing for this. Testing for heat stability required that the vaccine being tested be placed in an incubator at 40° C for four weeks. This was very time consuming and we therefore searched for a more rapid test. The available data was studied, and a comparison of heat stability results using both methods—the conventional method of four-weeks incubation and the desired method of one hour boiling—was done. It was found that many vaccine lots of higher initial potency passed the heat stability requirement of the boiling test, which was more stringent than the conventional test. However, there were exceptions: the vaccine that was in a vial, and certain vaccine lots produced by one manufacturer. In consultation with the WHO Collaborating Laboratories, the WHO eventually set up the procedures that required, first, a test using heat stability with boiling, failing which the vaccine could be retested using the standard incubation method of four weeks. The new procedures were first applied in 1969, having substantially reduced the testing time at a point when uninterrupted vaccine supply had been the critical problem. In the years that followed, almost 70 per cent of the test vaccines could meet the stability criteria applying the one hour boiling test, a good example of how the programme speeded up a simple idea with practical research and rapid decision.[4]

In the mid-1970s, the total amount of vaccine production in developing countries reached 150 million doses, or half of the global requirement. Some countries, like Kenya, even donated their vaccine to the programme in neighbouring countries in East Africa. Later, some of these countries were able to go on to produce other vaccines such as DPT (Diphtheria, Pertussis and Tetanus combined vaccine), OPV (Oral Polio Vaccine) and the measles vaccine, with bilateral assistance from organisations like the Japan International Cooperation Agency (JICA).

Improvements in Vaccination Technique

In 1969, I was participating in a mass smallpox vaccination campaign in a rural area of Bangladesh. Before noon, 20,000 people were already gathering to be ready for vaccinations using jet injectors. Bangladesh is a country with a high population density, among the world's highest. Similar conditions are found in northern

[4] I. Arita, "The Control of Vaccine Quality in the Smallpox Eradication Programme".

India, where advanced ancient civilisations developed along the Ganges River, leading to an increased population and higher population density. Unfortunately, these previously advanced areas had underdeveloped conditions and health services at the time of smallpox eradication, thus providing favourable conditions for the spread of communicable diseases like endemic cholera and smallpox. At the time, considering the conditions in Bangladesh, our vaccination team thought it most appropriate to use jet injectors for smallpox eradication mass vaccination campaigns. With two jet injectors, we were confident we could cover all the people in a single day. However, we soon realised that both the jet injectors had developed mechanical problems. Hastily, the repair manual was opened and we tried to fix the jet injectors. After two hours of failed effort we had to abandon the vaccination plan, with due apologies to the crowd of people who had been waiting to be vaccinated.

On another occasion, while I was visiting an Indian village in the early days of the programme, a young mother came to me with her child of three or four years of age. There was a lesion on the child's arm that looked like a severe bacterial infection following smallpox vaccination with a rotary lancet, a fearsome vaccination instrument used at the time in the Indian programme. On inquiring, my suspicions were confirmed. The mother asked for help, but I could do nothing except to clean and disinfect the lesion.

These two incidents suggested that for successful mass vaccination campaigns we needed a vaccination tool that was effective, but simpler and less harmful. Here, we were extremely lucky. In 1961, Benjamin Rubin of Wyeth Laboratories developed and patented a bifurcated needle as an innovative and effective method for vaccination (see figure 7.2). Subsequently, it was this method that was licensed for smallpox vaccination in the US. Upon learning this, D. A. Henderson specifically recommended that this new method be used for the eradication programme. Thus the bifurcated needle eventually became the main method for vaccination used by the programme. Henderson's recommendation for this needle is important as long as there is a risk of smallpox returning, which would require vaccination.

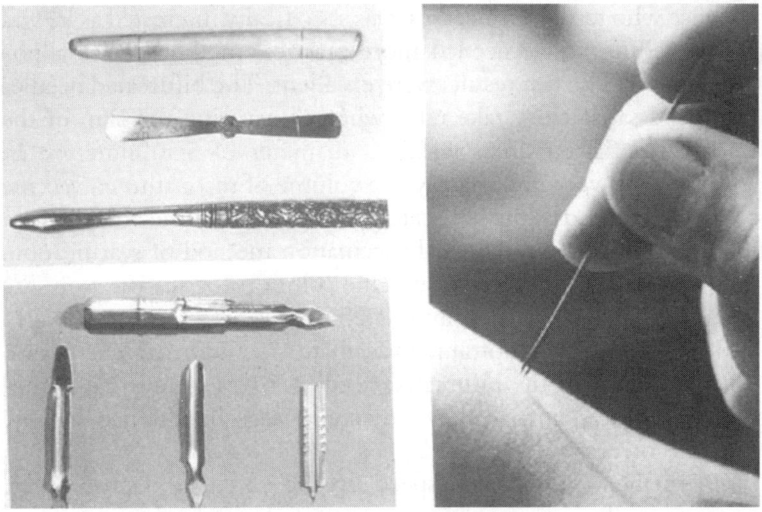

FIGURE 7.2 Various older vaccination devices and the bifurcated needle

Source: World Health Organization.

The history of the development of the bifurcated needle is indeed interesting. According to Rubin:

> I got an idea that if we cut a half of the pinhole in a point of a sewing machine needle, and sharpened the two points of the hole thus produced and then put this needle into reconstituted vaccine solution, the vaccine will be maintained in the space between the two points. If we then inserted the two needle points into skin, we could inoculate the vaccine into the skin.[5]

In fact, Rubin's idea worked very well, causing a good take (a vaccine pustule) from the vaccine virus to enter the skin. The vaccine pustule is a sign that the vaccination has induced immunity in the vaccinee. Wyeth had already obtained a production license from the US Food and Drug Administration (FDA) for a package containing a vaccine vial, reconstituted fluid and a tube containing 100 bifurcated needles. WHO sent the product to their smallpox field staff asking them to try it. A WHO colleague, Eshan Shafa, one

[5] I. Arita, *Smallpox Eradication: Target Zero* (Japan: Mainichi Press, 1979).

of those who tested the needles, was specifically interested as he was always telling us we needed more practical methods of smallpox vaccination. The test results were excellent. The bifurcated needles produced satisfactory take rates when puncturing the skin of the upper arm fifteen times within a diameter of 5 millimetres. In addition, and very importantly, the volume of reconstituted vaccine solution required by the bifurcated needle was only one-fourth of the volume required by the usual vaccination method of scarification. Instead of 0.01 millilitres of vaccine solution for scarification, the bifurcated needle used only 0.0025 millilitres. The studies also looked at how easily untrained vaccinators could be trained to give vaccinations with the bifurcated needle. It was found that within twenty minutes, virtually anybody could learn how to use the new needles correctly.

To further simplify and speed up the vaccination procedures, testing was done to compare the rate of skin infections for those vaccinated without cleaning the skin and those after cleaning. The results showed that cleaning the skin did not have an important effect on the infection rate, and after this practical study skin cleaning with alcohol or water before vaccination was omitted. In addition, special plastic containers, similar to toothpick dispensers, were developed and produced to accommodate 200 bifurcated needles in each tube which could then be easily dispensed during vaccination and also boiled in the container for sterilization.

All these innovations were tested during the actual field immunisation programmes, for specific periods of time. Finally, having confirmed the efficacy and efficiency of these innovations from results in the field, it was decided to set them as the standard vaccination method for the intensified smallpox eradication programme. Notably, Wyeth Laboratories made a generous contribution to WHO by not charging a patent fee for producing the bifurcated needles, as long as they were used for the WHO intensified smallpox eradication programme. WHO proposed the bid and selected a German producer to manufacture the needles owing to their superior quality steel, and their competitive pricing. Since 1969—when the new method started to be used widely for the global programme—it is estimated that roughly 50 million needles have been distributed.

Now, in the post-eradication era, the bifurcated needle is still the generally accepted smallpox vaccination method in the prevention or containment of smallpox transmission due to the deliberate or erroneous release of the smallpox virus, if it were to occur. Under such a circumstance, what would be the number of punctures required for the bifurcated needle method? This issue has been debated and decisions arrived at. For example, are three punctures for primary vaccination enough? I believe that fifteen punctures for both primary and revaccination (employed for successful containment during the smallpox eradication vaccination campaigns) would be a practical and effective method, as shown by more than a billion vaccinations of people of all ages. Also, if we do need smallpox vaccinations in future, it would be in a genuine emergency situation, requiring fully and absolutely assured efficacy from every vaccination given, even by rapidly trained staff members of less experience.

8

Evolution in Thinking

The New Strategy in India: A Crucial Stage

By 1973, the world map of smallpox-infected countries had altered greatly. Of the 135,000 cases of smallpox, 95 per cent were in only three countries, namely India, Pakistan and Bangladesh.

D. A. Henderson and I were talking in the WHO Smallpox Eradication Unit office in Geneva in June 1973. Through the office window, the white top of Mont Blanc was clearly visible. "The eradication programme is now at a critical stage", remarked Henderson. "Yes, it appears only difficult countries remain heavily endemic", I said. "Their containment strategy has shown its limits; with mass campaigns aiming at 100 per cent coverage unable to stop the transmission. Indian programme officers who worked with me in Uttar Pradesh accept the presence of smallpox cases in a village, but if they find an unvaccinated person they apologise as if they have made a great mistake. It seems that, paradoxically, 100 per cent vaccination is the purpose of the programme, and elimination of smallpox outbreaks has been forgotten. A drastic revision of strategy is necessary".[1]

We agreed, and began serious discussions on how to seek a breakthrough. My three-month experience in a district in northern India was a good subject to begin with.

> Arita: Judging from the results of active searches for smallpox cases in Muzzafarnagar district, Uttar Pradesh, it is feasible for health centre staff to visit all the villages if they stop their office work for one week in every month. During the visit they can make an active search for smallpox cases (reported and unreported). In this way special active searches can be organised to discover and list the actual number of cases. Subsequently,

[1] Personal conversation.

other teams can visit the infected villages with the intent of vaccinating households near the infected house.[2]

Henderson: Why don't we carry out this method in all of India?

Finally, we decided to try this method across the country. We also felt that the Indian government was greatly concerned about the lack of progress of the smallpox programme.

It is interesting to note here that Vladimir Zigmund, a Czechoslovakian WHO medical officer, was working for smallpox eradication in the state of Orissa in India at the time, and he too had in mind a similar approach on how to strengthen surveillance and containment of smallpox in India.

In addition to a different strategy, we also needed to brand the new WHO plan with a memorable phrase. A poster, indicating briefly the aim, was therefore necessary. We decided on "Target Zero" as the catch phrase.

However, one question remained. Would the Indian government accept such a drastic change in strategy? I recall a story I had heard. During the WHA in May 1973, India acknowledged the urgency of improving their smallpox eradication work, recognising that smallpox was already eradicated in Western Africa, with the last case in Nigeria being reported in 1970, while India reported more than 27,000 cases in 1972. During the plenary session of the 1973 WHA, when India proposed their cooperation to African nations to help their health programmes, one West Africa delegate asked the following question: "Can a nation, being unable to eradicate smallpox, help the nation already having eradicated smallpox?" The then prime minister, Indira Gandhi, was aware of this situation, and under her instructions the government was very keen to urgently improve the situation.

It is useful to mention here that the timing of mid-1973 was auspicious, as there were several extraordinary WHO smallpox eradication officers working in the WHO local office in India at the time. In addition to Nicole Grasset and William Foege, there were other hardworking smallpox officers like Zdeno Jezek (nicknamed "the dynamo"), of the Epidemiological Institute of

[2] Personal conversation.

Prague, Czechoslovakia, and Larry Brilliant, a young American doctor who was studying at an ashram in India. In fact, while at the ashram, it was Brilliant's guru who instructed him to go to WHO in New Delhi to meet a man from Japan and work for the WHO Smallpox Eradication Programme. I did not verify the truth of this story; however, there is a similar tale about the guru's prediction in relation to the smallpox programme. Eventually, after several unsuccessful attempts to join the programme during visits to the WHO office in New Delhi, Brilliant was finally accepted, and went on to play an important role in the fight to achieve "Target Zero".

After we had communicated our ideas about the new strategy to the Indian government, details of the plan were worked out in July 1973, in the meeting room of the WHO South-East Asia Regional Office (SEARO). The strategy was called the "Smallpox Eradication Intensified Search and Containment Strategy", in brief, the "Autumn Campaign: Surveillance and Containment". I was most happy to participate and assist in the meeting from Geneva.

At the meeting it was pointed out that the plan lacked a strategy for urban areas. It was therefore suggested that the period of July–August be utilised to scour the urban areas for incidences of smallpox, as the three-month monsoon made it impossible to navigate the villages due to the muddy dirt tracks. The suggestion was well received and quickly agreed upon.

> OK, let us immediately put the plan into execution in towns of more than five hundred thousand people.
>
> As soon as the rainy season ends, the state governments can execute the intensified strategy. With this new strategy, public health workers will visit certain assigned villages for a week in a month, while stopping their routine work to engage in searching for smallpox cases.
>
> As part of the strategy, before visiting households, workers can first ask village chiefs, elders and religious leaders about the presence or absence of smallpox cases. They can also ask about cases at local tea stalls and restaurants, as well as elementary school teachers, while walking through the villages. A village can be divided into four sections, east, west, north and south. With at least two or three family members asked about the presence or absence of cases in each section, examination of all village residents is not necessary.

At the meeting it was further decided that:

> A containment team would be put at each health centre and dispensary. If a case were found in a village, the containment team would carry out vaccinations in the infected village to prevent the spread of the disease. The target for this strategy would be to achieve "zero number of smallpox endemic villages". With the emphasis on number of cases, it was seen as essential to collect information on the number of villages with outbreaks and containment at the end of each week.

The following was finally agreed upon:

> That the new strategy would be first started in the states of Uttar Pradesh, Bihar, Madhya Pradesh and West Bengal, where the largest epidemics were occurring. Following our experience in these four states, the strategy would then be expanded to cover the rest of India.[3]

Following this meeting, the WHO programme officers prepared an action plan to implement the new strategy, in consultation with Indian national programme officers. Record-keeping was considered a high priority, with survey forms required. The challenge lay in including all the necessary information, while keeping the form simple. Two separate forms were developed, one for the supervisors and one for the workers who carried out the search for smallpox cases.

After the basic containment strategy was accepted, the next step involved agreeing on the extent of vaccination coverage in the infected villages. For instance, should only the houses around the smallpox case be vaccinated, or should the entire infected village and/or also the nearest neighbouring villages be vaccinated? Based on the programme experiences in West Africa and elsewhere, it was recommended that about fifty houses, I repeat, only 50 houses, surrounding the infected house should be the standard size for containment vaccination. This was in fact a revolutionary new strategy in India, which, in retrospect, was the correct recommendation as it worked very well.

Another difficult question involved how to deal with the cases found during the search. In India, in the past, smallpox isolation wards were usually set up, with the result that actual smallpox cases were at times placed together with suspected smallpox cases and

[3] Arita, *Smallpox Eradication*.

chickenpox cases. This had the unhappy, negative effect of non-smallpox cases being infected by the virus and further disseminating smallpox on their return home. It was therefore agreed that home isolations with a house guard would be the best solution. A house guard would be employed from the same village to prevent people moving in and out of the infected home, and to prevent smallpox cases from leaving the house.

It was further decided that the standard indicator of the termination of transmission in a village, which would allow the closing of an outbreak, would be a continuous six-week period without new cases of smallpox. In this way, villages where no new smallpox cases were found for six weeks would be removed from the list of endemic villages. This indicator would allow monitoring of the progress of the programme, showing the number of villages that had stopped transmission, and this result could then be compared with number villages that had not been successful in stopping transmission of smallpox. In a similar manner, other details of the implementation practices to put the strategy into effect were worked out.

Implementation guidelines, comprising the results of the aforesaid discussions, were printed and distributed to each of the states and districts of India. It was determined that the WHO headquarters in New Delhi would direct and assess the activity of each state, establishing a control structure with which to wage an all-out battle against smallpox.

Indira Gandhi, the then prime minister, also sent a letter with her signature to all district chiefs indicating that smallpox eradication was a top priority for the Government of India. The letter included the statement that it was not possible to accept that people will die unnecessarily of smallpox, and that each district chief should make strenuous efforts to eradicate the disease.

India's Miraculous Campaign and Target Zero

The result of the new smallpox campaign and "Target Zero" was quite dramatic.

The intensive active search for cases was carried out in the forty-third week of 1973 (see figure 8.1). That is, the staff at health centres in each state conducted an active search for smallpox cases for one week by stopping their routine work in the health centres. As a result, the number of cases detected increased suddenly from 800 in the forty-second week to more than 10,000 for the forty-third week. This means, only eight cases were reported in each 100 cases occurring in the endemic areas. Indeed, the surveillance teams, as well as the containment teams, were very busy conducting the search for hidden cases and containment vaccinations surrounding the cases detected, as planned.

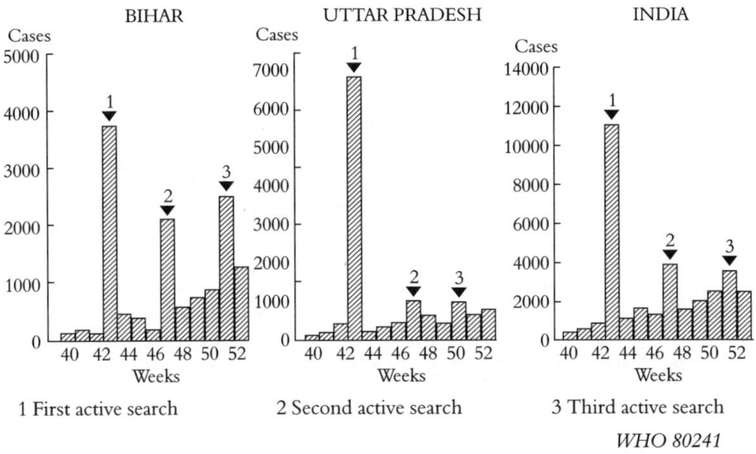

FIGURE 8.1 Impact of active searches on reporting of smallpox, India, 1973

Source: World Health Organization.[4]

At the time that the new smallpox eradication strategy was introduced, the number of international WHO smallpox officers, including short-term consultants, working in India was increased. The total number of international staff thus went up from thirteen in 1973, to thirty-three in 1974 and forty-six in 1975. The Indian government also assigned roughly the same number of young Indian health officers to the eradication programme. Supplies were

4 World Health Organization, *Final Report of the Global Commission for the Certification of Smallpox Eradication* (WHO, 1980), 44.

provided to implement the new strategy, with a total of 350 cars and about three million bifurcated needles for vaccination. As seen from the graph (figure 8.2), the number of cases per week increased sharply each time an active search was carried out from 1973 to 1974. However, the strengthened containment actions that followed the searches gradually improved in the latter half of 1974, leading to a sharp decline in cases.

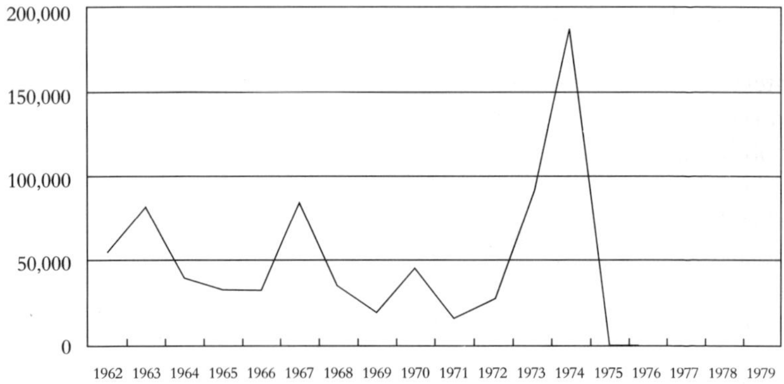

FIGURE 8.2 Number of smallpox cases reported by year: India

Note: Sharp incidence increase in 1973 and 1974.

Source: World Health Organization.

On 24 May 1975, about eighteen months following the introduction of the new active search and containment strategy, the last smallpox case in India occurred. A female beggar, 30-year old Saiban Bibi, had a rash in Assam state, in north-east India. The rash started while she was living on the platform of the railway station at Karimganj in Assam, after returning from Bangladesh. The case was promptly diagnosed as smallpox by the health officer, and containment carried out. Saiban Bibi recovered and went down in history as the last case of smallpox in India, with the source of the infection in Bangladesh.

During this accelerated special campaign in India, I often flew from Geneva to join the intensified campaign activities. At first, I was responsible, on behalf of WHO, to assist the operations in

West Bengal. Since September 1973, I had visited Calcutta (capital of West Bengal) several times. One night, in the hotel, following the first special active search, I was really moved to hear about the large increase in smallpox cases to 10,000 after the first search was completed in the forty-third week. These figures indicated the weak disease surveillance system that had been prevalent and the extent of under-reporting of cases in India at the time. However, we understood that once we located every source of the infection, that is every outbreak, then containment to get rid of the virus could be carried out. This eventually proved to be the case, with India interrupting the transmission of the smallpox virus in May 1975, within eighteen months from the implementation of the special mobilisation strategy.

I quote here a statement made by Indira Gandhi on 30 July 1975, celebrating the absence of cases for more than six weeks throughout India. She said, "Smallpox is a disease of economic backwardness.... It is important to ensure that there is no relapse through complacence or negligence. Our vigilance must continue".

To me, the principal lessons of this victory over smallpox are twofold. First, any critical health programme, limited by time, requires the correct strategy based on adequate research. In the case of smallpox eradication, it was the surveillance/containment strategy, first developed and implemented effectively by the smallpox eradication programme in West Africa. Second, such a strategy was effectively implemented at the global level, by all nations with continuing smallpox transmission, without any exception due to economic, social or political factors. In the case of India, it is commendable that the country's health services finally abandoned the traditional belief that 100 per cent vaccination theoretically stops the smallpox transmission, and shifted gears to the new autumn campaign with extraordinary efficacy. Although it was late development, it was still an extraordinary success in the population of 550 million, the world's largest population next to China. Table 8.1 gives the number of smallpox cases across India from 1973 to 1976. Figure 8.3 shows the poster proclaiming reward for smallpox cases in India.

TABLE 8.1 Smallpox cases, all India, 1973–76.

Year	*Number of Cases*
1973	88,114
1974	198,003
1975	1,436
1976	0

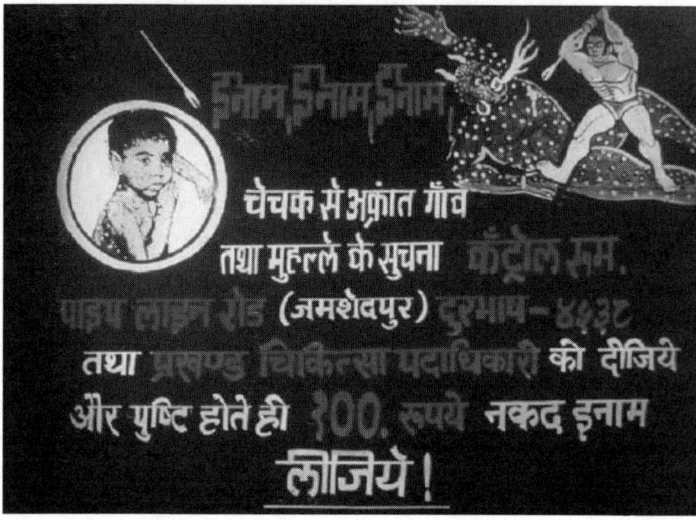
इनाम, इनाम, इनाम
चेचक से अक्रांत गाँव
तथा मुहल्ले के सुचना
(जमशेदपुर)
तथा
को दीजिये
और पुष्टि होते ही 100. रुपये नकद इनाम
लीजिये !

FIGURE 8.3 Poster proclaiming reward for reporting smallpox cases, India

Source: World Health Organization.

A few health experts in the West termed the campaign a miracle (see figure 8.3). Historical and administrative documentation of the Indian programme is available in detail in the books by Larry Brilliant and Sanjoy Bhattacharya.[5]

[5] R. N. Basu, Z. Jezek and N. A. Ward, *The Eradication of Smallpox from India* (New Delhi: WHO South-East Asia Regional Office, 1979); Sanjoy Bhattacharya, *Expunging Variola: The Control and Eradication of Smallpox in India 1947–1977* (Hyderabad: Orient Longman, 2006); L. Brilliant, *The Management of Smallpox Eradication in India* (Michigan: The University of Michigan Press, 1985).

Campaign in West Bengal

I describe here my observations of the operations in West Bengal, a state with a population of fifty million people. Present-day Calcutta, the capital city, is best described as a mix of varied influences. It is as well known for its heavily crowded slums, as it is for the famous mountainous Darjeeling district, located in the north of the state. In fact, Darjeeling boasts its very own home-grown celebrity, Sherpa Tenzing Norgay, who accompanied Edmund Hillary, one of the first people in history to finally reach the summit of Everest. So, it was with great joy that I could, with the purpose of searching for smallpox cases, also visit Darjeeling twice, in addition to the Calcutta slums. The sight of the great Mt Kanchenjunga towering at over 8,000 metres, against a rich blue sky, has always been for me a sight to behold.

In West Bengal, 18,496 smallpox cases were found in 1973, 11,094 in 1974, 124 in 1975, and zero in 1976. The scale of the epidemic was next to that of the states of Uttar Pradesh and Bihar. The State Health Office organised thirteen containment teams, and deployed them to each district for the containment of smallpox outbreaks. Additionally, they were joined by four to five WHO smallpox officers from outside the state. Once every month, all the teams gathered in Calcutta to exchange information and discuss the strategy for the next month.

I narrate here an amusing anecdote about one WHO officer which simply proves that even among the organisation's officers there were those who were far from perfect. One day, while in Calcuta, I received a telegram from a WHO officer stating that he had found three smallpox infected villages in the northern part of the state. The government records showed that the village did not have any smallpox outbreaks. Had a new outbreak occurred? The health office of the West Bengal government was very concerned about this matter, and I immediately set out to confirm the report myself. Three days were spent on the trip, only to discover that all of the three reported cases were actually chickenpox, and not smallpox. I was relieved, for I had feared that the transmission of the smallpox virus had continued. However, the entire episode had put WHO in bad light. It meant that a WHO epidemiologist had misdiagnosed the cases. At the end of this trip, I happened to meet the officer who had caused all the trouble. However, the arrows of criticism that I had prepared to fire at him were dispersed like mist when I finally met him. On the day of our meeting, I faced the man across a river about 20 metres wide. The officer began to cross the river to come to me by riding on the back of a water buffalo, borrowed from a villager. However, the buffalo began to slowly and comfortably crouch down in the middle of the river to enjoy the cooling water. Of course, the offending officer, who was on the back of the buffalo, also began to sink in the water right in front of my eyes. When I saw the man thoroughly wet when he at last dragged himself on to the land, I could not be so strict. I told him briefly that all three of the cases were chickenpox, and comforted him by telling that even a good epidemiologist could make a mistake.

I end this chapter with an interesting insight into human behaviour vis-à-vis smallpox during the eradication era, over thirty years ago. Very often, variola was misdiagnosed; at times this was done inadvertently, and at times deliberately. The former was due to poor technical knowledge or carelessness, while the latter was purely out of selfish interests.

At times, it is these selfish interests that kept the smallpox reports hidden from national governments and health centres. Reports that wrongly reduced the number of smallpox cases (or even reported zero cases) gravely misguided the programme strategy. Eventually, of course, the eradication efforts overcame this serious defect through training as well as rewards to reporters.

The incorrect diagnosis of smallpox during that time reminds me of the following words of French philosopher Baron de Montesquieu (1689–1755): "Ce n'est pas l'esprit qui fait les opinions c'est le coeur" (Your opinions are not dictated by your mind, but by your heart).

9

The Final Battle in Bangladesh: Victory in Asia

As the number of smallpox cases lessened, the WHO smallpox officers started a raffle to guess the date of the onset of the final case in each country. Questions of the following nature were commonplace:

> When will we see the final case in India?
> When will we see the final case in Bangladesh?
> When will we see the final case in the world?

A $5 bill, together with a piece of paper with the year, month and day written on it, was collected from everyone, sealed and kept in a safe. It was decided that the safe would be opened when the last smallpox case was declared, with the winner being the one with the closest date. We were certain that someone would collect the prize money, although I forget now who won the raffle. However, there were dramatic swings in the progress of smallpox eradication in Bangladesh from 1970 to 1975, making it very difficult guess the date of the last case. The fortunes of the programme alternated from optimistic to pessimistic, with the cases lessening to very low levels and then increasing as outbreaks swept the country. Finally, after all the outbreaks were contained, the person who had chosen the most optimistic date for the last case won.

Bangladesh reported zero cases in 1971, as shown in figures 9.1 and 9.2. Then in 1972, there were huge outbreaks, with 10,754 cases reported. This large swing in the number of cases demonstrates how the programme strategy and war altered the progress of smallpox eradication.

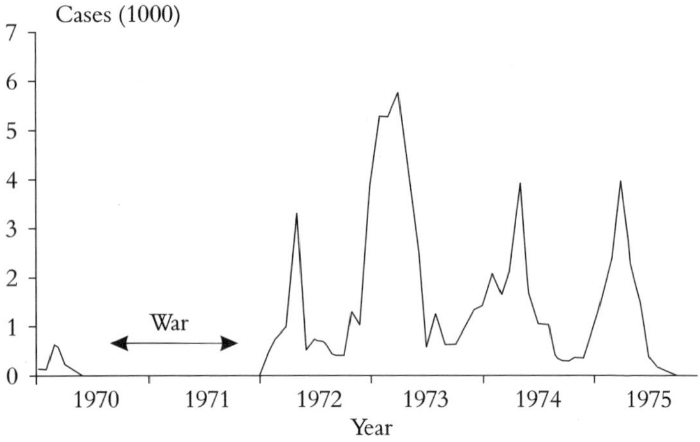

FIGURE 9.1 Number of smallpox cases by month, Bangladesh

Source: World Health Organization.

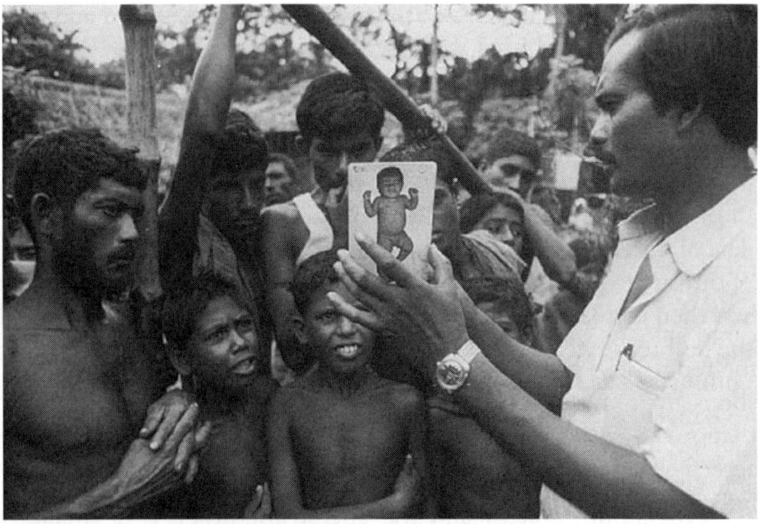

FIGURE 9.2 A surveillance team member holding a recognition card questions villagers in Bangladesh

Source: World Health Organization.

In spring 1970, I was in East Pakistan (now called Bangladesh) where we found smallpox transmission progressing only in the north, with no cases reported in the south. The programme's meticulous and active search for cases verified the reported figures. We discussed whether to alter our strategy from the then ongoing nation-wide mass vaccination campaign to surveillance and containment measures, with all the programme resources moved to the north. After serious discussion, everyone, including the Bangladesh national smallpox eradication staff, agreed to change the strategy. Thus the surveillance and containment strategy was started in Bangladesh. In retrospect, it was an excellent move. The new operation was started during the spring and early summer, when smallpox transmission rates increase. The smallpox transmission rate begins to drop with the start of the summer rains. The new campaign made surprisingly rapid progress, with no smallpox cases discovered from September 1970 to March 1971 despite continuing active surveillance. The new strategy was a huge success (see figure 9.2).

Then, disaster struck. The Indo-Pakistan war started, with East Pakistan as the main battlefield. The war led to the interruption of all smallpox eradication activities, from March to December 1971. The war ended in December 1971, with no smallpox cases being reported from the newly independent Bangladesh. I personally believe that Bangladesh was free of smallpox transmission from April to December 1971.

I returned to Bangladesh in January 1972, at a time when a massive movement of refugees was underway; they were returning from refugee camps in India, most notably from the smallpox infected camp at Salt Lake in West Bengal. The capital, Dhaka, contained the remnants of the war, with broken cars left in the streets, closed shops and food shortages causing famine. The office of the United Nations Disaster Relief Organization (UNDRO) had kindly agreed to let me join their helicopter flights to visit all the smallpox infected or at-risk areas. The smallpox cases among the returning refugees resulted in the re-introduction of the disease and its spread throughout Bangladesh. I met M. M. Hoque, the then minister of health, in his office. He welcomed me with a terse "I am not happy to see you because you always come to me when smallpox is epidemic in my country", although his eyes showed he was joking. "I sent smallpox teams with boats throughout the Ganges delta to fight the epidemics," he informed me, "but it was difficult and too late, and we failed to stop the spread". As shown in the figure 9.1, 10,700 smallpox cases were eventually reported in 1972.

I left Bangladesh in late spring of 1972, when Stanley Foster, a CDC epidemiologist from USA, arrived to replace me. Stan had previously worked in the West Africa Smallpox Eradication Programme. He made a great contribution to the fight there, one of the most difficult areas covered in the global eradication programme. Stan remained in Bangladesh for three years, until the discovery of the last smallpox case in November 1975.

Last Battle in Asia

Imagine working in Bangladesh during the summer of 1973, without knowing the events that would unfold in 1974 and 1975. The epidemic curve showed an abrupt decline from 6,000 cases in May, to 700 in July. Many expected that the number of cases would continue to decline to near zero by August or September 1973. However, the opposite happened. There was another increase in smallpox cases, with the number of cases in September 1974 still around 500 per month. Could target zero ever be reached? The total number of cases still added up to 16,485 in 1974. In fact, strangely enough, as the number of smallpox cases inched closer to zero, there would be a sudden increase in the incidence of smallpox. This led some pessimists to say that the effort was hopeless, as the same increase in cases was repeated every year. Nevertheless, the staff remained optimistic and a new emergency eradication plan was prepared together with the government. The number of international WHO operations officers was doubled: from six in 1973 to twelve in 1974. Then, as the situation was improving again, the government started to demolish the slums of Dhaka. This resulted in a large number of people, including smallpox patients, losing their homes and being forced to leave, scattering in all directions to all parts of the country. Yet again the number of smallpox cases increased dramatically with this single act. In February 1975, the president of Bangladesh declared "a state of smallpox emergency". The WHO Bangladesh programme officers were increased to thirty and additional health workers were mobilised.

The infection peaked in April 1975, with 4,500 cases being reported during the month, almost the same as when the numbers peaked in May 1974. However, after April 1975, the number of cases declined steadily.

Barisal district lies in the southern part of Bangladesh, at the mouth of the Ganges River, an area with many islands separated by large rivers. One of the administrative areas of Barisal district was Bhola sub-division, located on an island measuring about 130 kilometres from north to south and 20 kilometres in width from east to west. In 1975, Bhola was a very fertile rice-growing area, with a population of about one million. On 6 November 1975, a surveillance team searching for smallpox cases on Bhola Island received information that there was a smallpox case in Kuralia village. Investigations showed that the report was indeed correct and that a three-year old girl, Rahima Banu, would turn out to be the last case in Bangladesh (figure 9.3), with the date of onset of rash on 16 October. The last case in Bangladesh was also the last case of smallpox in Asia, and the last case of variola major (the most severe form of smallpox, killing up to thirty to forty of every 100 cases).

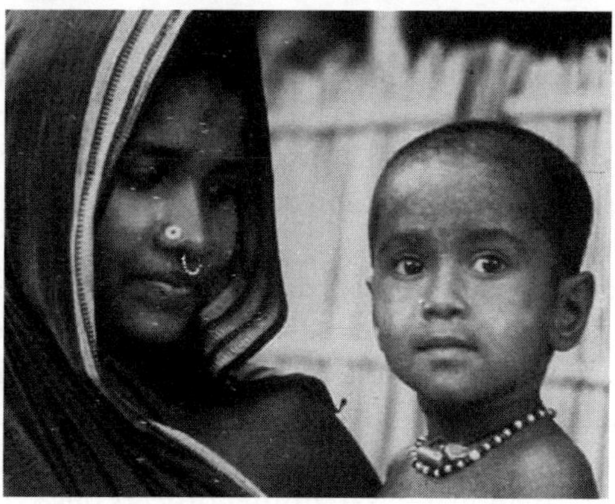

FIGURE 9.3 The last case of smallpox: Bangladesh

Source: World Health Organization.

Pakistan, Afghanistan and Nepal

The WHO-assisted smallpox eradication programme was also intensified in Pakistan in 1973, following the development of the plan for all-out mobilisation for surveillance and containment in the Asian subcontinent. The programme made rapid progress in Pakistan, reaching zero in 1974, one year earlier than India and Bangladesh. The last case in Pakistan occurred in Punjab province, in the northern part of the country, with onset of rash on 6 October 1974.

In Nepal, the smallpox eradication strategy was closely coordinated with the strategy followed in India. This was primarily because there were large population centres concentrated in the terai, the flatlands bordering India. The frequent movement of people between this area and the northern India states of Bihar and Uttar Pradesh led to many outbreaks of smallpox. Considering the heavy traffic across the border, the spillover of outbreaks to Nepal could be expected, and they would never cease as long as outbreaks continued in Bihar and Uttar Pradesh. The eradication programme in Nepal was successful in containing the importations of smallpox and was able to record its last case in April 1975, one month before the last case of smallpox in India.

Similarly, in Afghanistan, the smallpox eradication programme progressed well, with interrupted endemic transmission in 1972, and containment of the last imported case from Pakistan in 1973. However, the variolation, as in Africa, posed a problem for the smallpox "end game". It had been a practice from ancient times in Afghanistan. From 1970 to 1973, smallpox was reported from 237 villages, with about 20 per cent of these outbreaks thought to be caused by this variolation.

Fortunately, as smallpox cases decreased, the source of variolation materials became scarce, and finally disappeared, with the exception of materials stored by variolators in cold climates. It was found that with the loss of new smallpox materials, the stored specimens eventually lost their viability in due course and could no longer infect people. National programme officers also offered small gold-coloured containers to the variolators so that the programme staff could track the specimens. This made it easier to destroy the stocks of materials. The ending of smallpox transmission also ended the source of the variolators' materials and the threat of smallpox outbreaks from this source.

This is a very brief summary of some key points on how smallpox eradication was achieved in Asia. In the next chapter, we turn to the situation in Africa, the location of the last remaining smallpox cases.

10

Fight in the Horn of Africa

In Africa, following the successful smallpox eradication efforts in West and Central Africa, countries in the eastern and southern parts of the continent also carried out relatively effective smallpox eradication campaigns. In fact, by 1973, all the formerly smallpox endemic countries in Africa had apparently interrupted transmission with exception of the four countries in the Horn of Africa (see table 10.1).

TABLE 10.1 Smallpox cases in selected sub-saharan African countries, 1973–79

	1973	1974	1975	1976	1977	1978	1979
Ethiopia	5,414	4,439	3,935	916*	-	-	-
Djibouti	14	13	-	-	-	-	-
Somalia	7	11	14	39*	3,229*	-	-
Kenya	-	4	-	-	5*	-	-
Others	-	-	-	-	-	-	-

Note: * indicates smallpox incidence detected by extensive surveillance and containment operations in the Horn of Africa.

Source: World Health Organization.

Djibouti succeeded in stopping smallpox transmission in 1974, leaving only three countries—Ethiopia, Somalia and Kenya—with smallpox cases in the Horn of Africa. Thus, on the whole, the epidemiological situation in Africa did look rather promising in 1974. In retrospect, the period of the 1960s and 1970s was quite favourable for the eradication effort. It was a period characterised by a newly optimistic political atmosphere, despite the Cold War, a time of peace after the Second World War, with newly independent African nations embracing fresh hope of being able to contribute to the happiness of their citizens. Perhaps, the positive atmosphere contributed to many new African nations deciding to contribute to this global humanistic initiative of disease eradication. From a more operational viewpoint, the successful West African smallpox eradication campaign may have also contributed to stimulating the participation of these countries throughout the region.

With this backdrop, in May 1976, participants at the WHA optimistically discussed the status of the global smallpox eradication effort. Nine years had elapsed since the start of the intensified programme in 1967. South America has not reported a single smallpox case in five years. In the Asian subcontinent, Bangladesh continued to maintain zero cases six months after the last case despite intensive searches for cases. In the African continent, smallpox had been restricted to Ethiopia, in the Horn of Africa. Achieving zero incidences of smallpox in Ethiopia could well mean the global eradication of the disease.

All eyes turned to the programme in Ethiopia. How was it progressing? In the beginning, the work had been difficult due to limited resources, as well as the extremely difficult communications in the mountainous areas and deserts of the country. However, efforts were improved, as additional resources were provided and the areas with continuing transmission were continually reduced. Nevertheless, the programme in Ethiopia had its share of doubters too. Many debated the truth behind the claim that barring Ethiopia smallpox had been eradicated in the subcontinent. They were reassured by the repeated WHO investigations, which revealed zero cases. On our part, we felt that the year to follow would be most critical to the programme.

The WHA passed resolution 29.54 concerning smallpox eradication in May 1976, and I quote here some crucial parts.

> Noting with satisfaction that smallpox is now restricted to only a few remote villages of a single country and that interruption of smallpox transmission is believed to be imminent.
>
> Congratulate the many countries which have made and are making such successful and determined efforts to eradicate smallpox.

The resolution continued to stress the importance of surveillance, laboratory investigation and international cooperation. It thus concluded:

> Request further the Director-General to undertake a study of the organization of a world conference on the problems of eradicating smallpox and to report on the subject to the Executive Board and to the Thirtieth WHA.

Parenthetically, my personal records of that period show that Somalia had reported five cases in January and February of 1976, but no cases from March to August.

After the WHA meeting, the smallpox eradication unit staff met in the smallpox office at WHO headquarters in Geneva, and exchanged comments and thoughts on the WHA discussions on smallpox eradication. D. A. Henderson commented:

> You know Babe Ruth, the famous homerun hitter. He is in the batter's box. He points out straight with his bat at the center field stands. He is saying that he will hit the ball there. The pitcher threw the ball. The white ball that Ruth hit flew straight like an arrow to the center field stands, and disappeared.
>
> The year of 1976 will be the tenth year of the 10-year program which started in 1967. The game would be in our hands. If the last case in the world could be recorded before the end of 1976, WHO would be the world's best homerun hitter for health!

We all laughed, remembering the efforts of the past ten years and the faces of our colleagues, both national and international, who had worked so hard and so well together. With great expectations of impending success, we raised and discussed various options to celebrate the successful end of the programme,

> It will be the completion of the 10-Year Program we proposed, right on schedule, won't it?
>
> How about sending telegrams to our friends in Bangladesh and India as follows:
>
> Zero cases in Ethiopia. WHO declares smallpox eradicated throughout the world within ten years as promised.

> How about opening bottles of champagne in Addis Ababa, Ethiopia and Dhaka, Bangladesh to celebrate managing to reach the last case in two continents, Asia and Africa? Taking into account a 5-hour time lapse, the champagne in a lunch party in Addis Ababa would correspond to the champagne in a great dinner party in Dhaka. [1]

The pleasant, relaxed atmosphere at the above meeting encouraged the entire smallpox staff at the WHO headquarters. However, our sense of elation was short-lived.

Initial Sign of Continued Smallpox Transmission in the Horn of Africa

Before we begin to discuss what happened in the Horn of Africa, I explain here the staffing pattern of the smallpox team at the WHO headquarters in Geneva, as the smallpox eradication programme entered the final phase of the fight in 1977. Since 1967, the programme had progressed in an environment of excellent teamwork, not only of the WHO staff, but also of the WHO consultants who had assisted the programme with keen professional and personal interest. However, at headquarters, D. A. Henderson, Ehsan Shafa (from Iran, who first worked at the WHO Regional Office for the Eastern Mediterranean) and I were the only three regular staff members who had worked together continuously in excellent harmony from the beginning of the programme.

In February 1977, Henderson, the chief of the global smallpox eradication unit at WHO, left Geneva for Baltimore (details given in chapter 4). Consequently, the smallpox team at the WHO headquarters was urgently rearranged. Ehsan Shafa remained, and was joined by Joel Breman from the CDC in Atlanta, USA, and Alexander Gromyko from the Epidemiological Institute in Moscow, formerly USSR. Both of them were excellent epidemiologists and had a good reputation among colleagues and international public health workers. Having replaced Henderson as chief of the unit, I assumed the task of achieving target zero globally, and continued in this position until the end of the programme. It was a position I was

[1] Personal conversations.

happy to fill, even though I was somewhat tired after many years of strenuous efforts; but the programme had to go on.

Tired or not, events in the Horn of Africa in late 1976 and 1977 were to provide a new test for me and the other smallpox staff that demanded urgent and strenuous action. But first, let us look more closely at the situation of the smallpox programme in the region called the Horn of Africa, which consists of all or parts of Ethiopia, Somalia, Djibouti, and Kenya.

11

Smallpox in Ethiopia

The smallpox eradication programme in Ethiopia started only in 1971. Globally, it was the last smallpox endemic country. At the time, Ethiopia was a target for aid from many Western countries. Denmark and Sweden focused their interest on strengthening the development of basic health services, while USA was supporting malaria eradication. It was said that one third of the national health budget was being used for malaria eradication. Under such a situation, the Ethiopian government appeared reluctant to initiate a national smallpox eradication programme as proposed by the WHO. However, the launch of the eradication programme in East Africa, including Sudan, Kenya and Uganda, contributed to the Ethiopian government's decision to join and start the eradication programme in 1971.

How to plan the programme was the key question. At the time, if WHO workers launched the programme via motorable roads, they would cover only 20 per cent of the total Ethiopian population. The remaining 80 per cent of the people who lived in the mountainous and desert areas would not be covered. To reach these areas, one needed to travel on the back of a donkey or camel, or walk. In addition, the number of health facilities was very limited, both in the rural provinces and urban areas. The few health facilities that existed engaged in public health and curative services, but served only a limited portion of the total population.

Thus, the programme was started by about a dozen Ethiopian sanitarians, or health inspectors, and about the same number of young US Peace Corps volunteers. Later on, Japanese and Austrian volunteers, as well as additional American Peace Corps volunteers, joined the programme. Two operations officers of the WHO were also assigned to the team. The WHO also supplied cars to enable implementation of the programme.

Box 11.1 People readily accepted vaccination in parts of Ethiopia

Alan Schnur, then a US Peace Corps volunteer working in the Ethiopia Smallpox Eradication Programme, personally encountered an interesting event in a village in Welega province, western Ethiopia, as he describes below:

In 1971, a two-man vaccination team arrived on the agreed day in a village, expecting to find around 100 people. Instead, they were surprised to find a huge crowd milling around, waiting for their arrival. It appeared that the people were aware of the smallpox cases in nearby areas, recognised the usefulness of smallpox vaccination and were eager to protect themselves and their families. The vaccination session was to be held in an open area around a simple government office, a rectangular hut with mud walls and a tin roof. There were limited prospects for crowd control. At first, the plan was to vaccinate inside the building, but with only one door it would not have been possible to create a flow of people. The two vaccination team members hurriedly conferred as to how to proceed. There was fear of a riot as people pushed to get vaccinated first; and the same result if the team did not vaccinate. The village elders were requested to maintain order as far as possible and to provide persons to control the crowd. One table was set up outside the building for the team members to work on. As the team members broke their vials of freeze-dried smallpox vaccine and added the diluents there was suddenly silence, like the quiet before the storm.

As the team started vaccinating with bifurcated needles, the people surged forward to be vaccinated. The people assigned to maintain order struggled gallantly, but were clearly fighting a losing battle. After two hours of frantic vaccinating, the crowd was still pushing forward and extending their arms to the vaccinators. The vaccinators grabbed the nearest extended arm and vaccinated in the required target area over the deltoid muscle on the upper arm. Finally, after four hours, the crowd started to thin out although there still remained a general lack of order. The vaccinators exchanged harried, but triumphant looks as it became more likely that the day would end with all the people vaccinated. By the end of five hours, only a few dozen people remained, with some new people coming as the crowd departed, ready to politely wait their turn, allowing the team to finish up at a much more leisurely pace.

At the end of the day, the team counted the containers with used needles. It turned out that more than 1,500 vaccinations had been provided, in rather chaotic circumstances, with no breaks taken until after the crowd had dispersed.

One of the key factors for a successful immunisation programme is the interest of the people in vaccination. Similar episodes were observed in some other countries with limited health resources in sub-Saharan Africa and South Asia and these greatly helped the development of the global programme. However, it should be noted that there was also strong resistance to immunisation in some areas.

The establishment of plans similar to those made in India and Bangladesh seemed to be quite impossible, although it was agreed that the strategy of surveillance and containment would be used from the beginning of the programme. It was decided that surveillance teams would be set up, and sent to each province. The search for cases in the interiors would mainly be done by walking, with as many vaccinations as possible done by the teams as and when they found cases. Although the villagers in the provinces where the work initially started accepted vaccination whole-heartedly, reaching the villagers in Ethiopia presented considerable difficulties. An example of a difficult field trip is well explained in a 1972 report by Russ Handzus, a young American Peace Corps volunteer working in Ilubabor province in south-west Ethiopia.

Russ and his team planned to look for smallpox cases while travelling about 180 miles from Gambella, through the hot flat bush country of south-western Ethiopia to the western-most point in Ethiopia. They left the town of Gambella on Thursday by Land Rover, but had to leave the car at Gilo River mission station because the river was getting too high to drive across. After intensive discussion, they finally decided to walk. Here, I reproduce some extracts from their diary:

> On Monday, 17 April 1972 the mission airplane landed at Gilo. We discussed with the pilot if he could pick us up from Tirgol, on the Sudan border, in about two weeks and take us back to Gilo. He said he could probably pick us up on Monday May 1st. He added, "If I'm not there by 8 am, then I'm not coming!"

We arranged for guides, who also carried our vaccine and bed rolls, and had lunch before Wassihun [Wassihun Wondemagegnehu, Sanitarian], myself and the rest of our team started walking at around 3 p.m., heading west to the Sudan border. Jack's [Jack Howard, US Peace Corps volunteer] team took off walking in a different direction the next morning with an interpreter and two guides who also served as porters. His trip was more difficult. He followed the Akobo River, which was almost completely dry. There were just a few muddy low spots here and there which served as their drinking and bathing water supply.

For all of us it was a long, hot walk. Day after day plodding or quickstepping through the western reaches of an area as far away from the comforts of civilization as any place on earth. However, there was also great natural beauty—in the cool sparkling mornings, the ever constant companionship of the Gilo River. It was very hot, but if we had enough water we did all right. I kept thinking that once you set yourself to do something, there's nothing to do but to do it.

Hunger was an occasional problem. The little food that we brought made a difference. About three cans of C-ration meat, a couple of candy bars, some sour candy, and a can of cheese. The Anuaks living in the villages generously shared their food with us. Usually sorghum porridge and a little fish stew. Some of the villages near Tirgol were experiencing famine because they had been cleaned out by the *Anyanya*, or South Sudanese rebels, many of whom came to Ethiopia to recuperate and regroup. However, the Anyanya were good to us. In fact they saved us several times. They gave us some bread and canned meat once when we had gone for about twenty hours without food. We marched with about 600 of them across a desert plain one day, shooting and carving up several antelope for our lunch and evening meals. As we met their different platoons throughout the wilderness we were intercepted, interrogated and had to show our WHO identity cards.

Late Thursday night, on the eleventh day out, we reached Tirgol. That day we had walked almost without stopping since 7:30 am. We found Jack in bed with severe dysentery. His party had arrived two nights before us. He had caught amoebic dysentery a few days before reaching Tirgol and became so weak that he thought he would die.

Monday morning, May 1st, Jack and I walked out to the runway. We sat on the wing of a wrecked DC-3 mapping mission plane there and waited. Our plane didn't come. The police sent out urgent messages on their radio set describing our condition. For two more days we languished, thinking that nobody in Gambella town or Mettu (the capital of Ilubabor) knew our plight.

> Wednesday morning came. We were sitting on our camp beds in the open air. Both of us were getting over our illnesses. Suddenly we were lifted from our lethargy by the drone of an airplane motor. We were so elated to hear the roar of the engine as it circled the town. It circled twice but then HEADED AWAY. My heart sank. Slowly it banked and came in low and landed. What a joy! God was with us. On take-off that little plane felt like a toy vibrating down the runway. But finally we gained speed and lifted off. We passed over the town and looked across the broad Pibor River into Sudan with a feeling of escape from a difficult place.

I would like to end this narrative with Russ's final comment.

> Whatever, we felt good that the job has been accomplished, with 6,000 people vaccinated against smallpox, thereby protecting a large stretch of the Ethiopia-Sudan border. I am thankful for the comradeship and moral support of Wassihun, my Ethiopian counterpart, without whom the campaign would have failed. [1]

In early 1970, I frequently visited Sudan and Ethiopia. One day, I flew from Khartoum to El Facher, a small border town situated in Darfur province in western Sudan, within the Sahara desert. I was going to investigate a report of smallpox cases, although I wondered at the time how smallpox could occur in such a sparsely populated area. On arrival, I found a small town with several shops selling hides and interesting silver coins containing the image of Maria Theresa, an Austrian queen of the eighteenth century. The town chief bid me to go to the town hall where some meeting was being held. There, I found a Swedish woman surrounded by about a dozen Arab men, discussing their trip in the Sahara desert. The woman was an anthropologist and she appeared to be talking with the men about the cultural behaviour of the nomads. They were quite helpful and during discussions confirmed that they had seen no sign of smallpox during their trips. Talking with them, and looking together at a map pointing out the route they had travelled, I felt that I could confirm that the smallpox reported from El Facher area was a false alarm. This was important information for the global eradication programme and for me. In the present day, such a trip

[1] From Russ Handzus' personal diary.

would be very difficult to undertake since this part of Sudan suffers from political unrest. How the world has changed!

Although these are just a few experiences of the smallpox eradication workers, they illustrate the difficulties which had to be overcome in some geographical areas, especially Ethiopia (see figure 11.1). Very clearly, the extreme dedication and special interest in reaching zero smallpox cases by the workers was the key. It is this spirit of the smallpox eradication staff that helped the Ethiopian programme achieve slow, but steady progress.

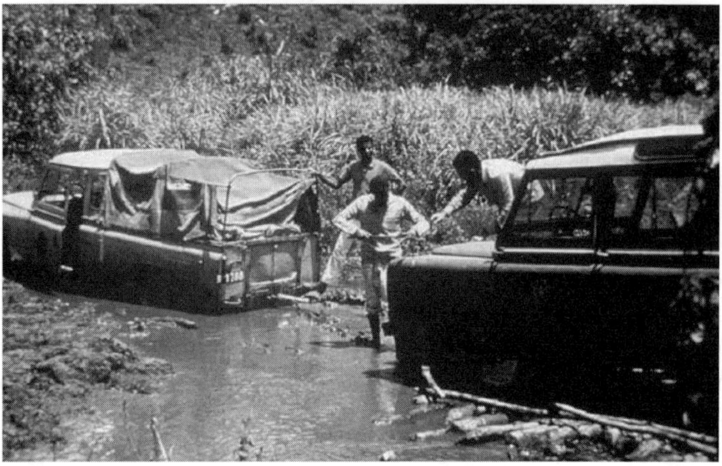

FIGURE 11.1 Programme vehicles bogged in Ethiopia

Source: World Health Organization.

When the programme started, surveillance was weak, with an average of 400–500 smallpox cases per year being reported throughout the country until 1970. It was also believed that these figures were greatly under-reported. Smallpox in Ethiopia was milder than in Asia, with only a 1 per cent case fatality rate, suggesting variola minor, which contributed to reduced reporting, as cases were not normally taken to hospitals or health facilities. In addition, variolation was also being practised in the country. As was found in Afghanistan, this practice enabled the spread of outbreaks. Since smallpox was well known to residents in the interior of the country, it was to be expected that the actual number of cases would be much higher. But the knowledge of smallpox among the local residents also meant that markets would be useful places to carry out surveillance activities since most people would recognise pictures of the disease. Table 11.1 shows the rapid success in interruption of transmission in Ethiopia, although much work was needed to verify that the cases had actually been reduced, through an intensive active search, if needed, using helicopters.

TABLE 11.1 Number of smallpox cases reported in Ethiopia, 1971–79

Year	Number of Cases
1971	26,329
1972	16,999
1973	5,414
1974	4,439
1975	3,935
1976	915
1977–79	0

Ato Yemane Tekeste was the national project manager in charge of the programme in Ethiopia as it neared completion. He was assisted by a few WHO officers and, as mentioned, by volunteers from several countries. Kurt Weithaler (Austria) was the first project director assigned by WHO to set up the smallpox eradication effort under the Ministry of Health. They all were dedicated workers with a keen interest in the programme, and without them Ethiopia would not have been freed from smallpox.

The regional interest to finish off the last foci of smallpox is illustrated by Sudan providing support for smallpox surveillance and vaccination in one *awraja* of the western province of Gojjam that bordered Sudan. In 1974, Sudan sent fourteen national health officers and three cars to Ethiopia to search for cases and carry out vaccination. In that year, USA also provided funds for renting two helicopters. In 1975, the programme activities were further strengthened, with four helicopters being used by the programme and the numbers of both WHO and Ethiopian programme officers being increased. By the end of 1975, smallpox was restricted to the northern highlands of the Gondar-Begemdir region and to the southern desert area of the Ogaden.

The last reported case of smallpox in Ethiopia occurred in the south-eastern desert area of the Ogaden, when a three-year-old girl named Amina Salat had onset of rash on 9 August 1976. The case was discovered at a small village called Dimo and was among sixteen outbreaks caused by variolation. After many years of heroic work, it appeared that target zero had finally been achieved. There was rejoicing all around, although at the time we knew that a lot of work still remained to make sure that there were no further unreported outbreaks.

I cannot end this chapter without acknowledging the contribution of a good friend, Dr Petrus Aswin Koswara, WHO medical officer (Indonesia), who died of heart attack during the work in Ethiopia in 1974, at the age of forty-three. His contribution to the programme was great, and included developing further the surveillance strategy for smallpox in the region. The difficult geographical conditions in Ethiopia may have been associated with this tragedy.

12

Somalia: The Beginnings of the Last Outbreaks in the Horn of Africa

Let us go back in time, to 27 September 1976. Seven weeks have elapsed since 9 August 1976, the date of the last smallpox case in Ethiopia. There have been no reports of any smallpox cases from Ethiopia or anywhere else in the world since. A first in the history of smallpox eradication: no active cases anywhere in the world.

And then, on 27 September 1976, I received a telephone call at nine o'clock in the evening at my home in Geneva from D.A. Henderson. He had in turn received a telephone report from the CDC, USA, which stated, "Particles like smallpox virus were observed through electron microscopy in a sample from Somalia". Henderson was hardworking, and his being in the office at that late hour was not unusual. Henderson continued,

> The sample is from smallpox suspects found in Somalia last week. Two patients with rash have been isolated in an infectious diseases quarantine station in Mogadishu. The first patient is an old woman, and the date of rash onset is 30 August. The second patient is a seventy-year old man, and the date of rash onset is 5 September. At first, the rash was considered to be chickenpox. However, with the progress of symptoms, the rash seemed unlikely to be chickenpox. The rash is rooted more deeply in the skin and its size was larger. Scab formation was abnormal and its surface was coarse and dirty. Because of these reasons, they urgently sent samples to the laboratory for analysis.[1]

At that point I was aware of the suspected smallpox case that was reported in Somalia a week earlier. I told Henderson that I would leave for Mogadishu by the earliest flight. "Everything depends on

[1] Author's notes.

the results of examination of the cases", I said. To which Henderson's reply was: "Yes, that should be the best way".

The problem was serious. Smallpox virus-like particles found by the electron microscope examination had not yet confirmed the cases as smallpox. Another three days were necessary before a definite diagnosis could be obtained by culturing the smallpox virus in eggs. However, I was unable to wait for the result, as I was to board the flight to Mogadishu the following day. Here, I would like to talk briefly about Somalia and the Ogaden desert.

The Ogaden Desert

The last case in Ethiopia occurred in the Ogaden desert, a wasteland extending over a large area from the southern region of Ethiopia to the north of Kenya and the north-west of Somalia. Two rivers run from the highlands of Ethiopia through the Ogaden desert, with tribes speaking the Somali language settled along the rivers. Besides the areas along the rivers, the desert is a wasteland of sand, rock and low shrubs. In this vast area, about 400,000 nomadic herdsmen roam (see figure 12.1), accompanying camels and goats in search of water and grass. It is believed that they walk up to 40 kilometres in a day when they hurry. The borderline between Ethiopia and Somalia is as clear as a ruled line on a map, but the nomadic herdsmen move back and forth across the border as if it does not exist.

What kind of country is Somalia? Somalia is located in the Horn of Africa, in the north-east region of the continent, with a population estimated at four million. The country borders the Ogaden desert of southern Ethiopia in the north, the desert in northern Kenya in the west and Djibouti in the east. It has a long coastline, 1,500 kilometres, stretching from the Red Sea to the Indian Ocean. Before gaining independence in 1960, the northern part of the country was an English colony while the southern part was governed by Italy. Therefore, while the national language is Somali, spoken by people throughout the country, there are many people in the south, including the capital Mogadishu, who can also speak Italian, in contrast to the people in the north who also speak English.

The Somalis are originally nomadic herdsmen. The Ogaden desert of Ethiopia and the wasteland of northern Kenya are now located in countries separate from Somalia, but nomadic Somali herdsmen freely walk across the borders. The people living on both sides of the country's borders—in Ethiopia and Kenya—and in the interior, all speak the Somali language and belong to the same tribes. Therefore, Somalia has historically claimed that the Ogaden desert is a part of Greater Somalia, in spite of internationally recognised boundaries. Ethiopia, on the other hand, has argued in favour of the current boundaries, while staking claim over part of the Ogaden desert, and viewing any outside claims to ownership of the land as a violation of her national sovereignty. These different views on ownership of the land have led to conflicts. In fact, the Somali tribes of the Ogaden (on the Ethiopian side of the border), organised a resistance movement called the Western Somalia Liberation Front, and initiated guerrilla activities in order to gain independence from Ethiopia. Somalia supported these activities.

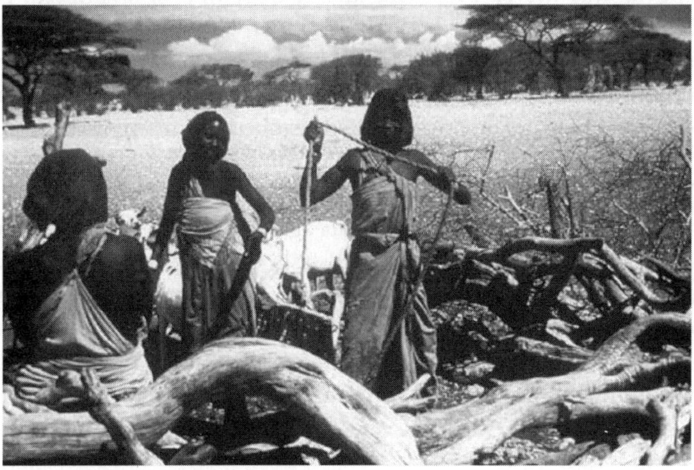

FIGURE 12.1 Nomad women in Somalia

Source: World Health Organization.

It was in the midst of such troubling circumstances, in August 1976, that an outbreak of smallpox was reported in Dimo village in

Ethiopia. The village had a population of sixty semi-settled nomadic herdsmen in Bale province.[2]

The flight between Geneva and Mogadishu is long, with a flight distance of about 7,500 kilometres. I departed from Geneva at half past six in the evening, and arrived at Rome at eight o'clock at night. There, I waited till one o'clock in the morning to board a Somali Airlines flight to Mogadishu. Thus, it took me about seven hours to fly from Rome to Mogadishu, including the stopover in Cairo. Looking around the airplane, I saw only twelve or thirteen passengers, all Somalians. Ever since Somalia had severed relations with the Western world to form an alliance with the Union of Soviet Socialist Republics (USSR) in 1972, visitors to Somalia for commerce and tourism were very few. Until March 1977, when Somalia ordered the deportation of all Soviet citizens, because of anger over its support of Ethiopia, the country was almost closed to the Western world.

Sitting in the dark Somali Airlines plane, various thoughts came to mind. Was the case of Mogadishu truly one of smallpox? Not necessarily. Experience had shown that several samples which initially showed smallpox virus-like particles, as observed by electron microscopy, later proved not to be smallpox at all. The reason being that the particles of vaccinia viruses cannot be distinguished from those of smallpox viruses by electron microscopy.

When suspected smallpox patient cases were found, health officers sometimes vaccinated these patients against smallpox. If the sample materials of patients had been carelessly obtained with vaccination needles, the sample materials could be contaminated with vaccinia viruses. There of course was the possibility that the sample materials from Mogadishu might be vaccinia viruses. However, at this stage, my thoughts on the matter were pure conjecture.

[2] For a discussion on the special geopolitical situation in the Horn of Africa, see R. Mansell Prothero, *The Sixth Melville Memorial Lecture* (Evanston: Northwestern University Press, 1968). The lecture was delivered under the auspices of the Program of African Studies, Northwestern University, on 9 October 1967. R. Mansell Prothero was then Reader in Geography at the University of Liverpool.

Supposing the cases were indeed smallpox, where was the source? Was there some correlation between the Ethiopian patients in the village of Dimo? Lets consider some facts. The distance from Dimo to Mogadishu is about 500 kilometres. This means that the outbreak in Mogadishu occurred one month after contact with patients of the village of Dimo. Usually, an outbreak of secondary cases occurs within about two weeks of contact. One month therefore was too long. Of course, there was a strong possibility that there might have been some undiscovered smallpox patients between the patients of Dimo and the patients of Mogadishu.

I also wondered about the vaccination situation in Somalia. During past six months, there had been no reports on the number of vaccinations given. At the time, there was only one WHO officer living in Somalia. Over the past four years, there had been about forty cases of imported smallpox into the country. Seven to fourteen smallpox cases were reported each year, from 1973 to 1975. In 1976, only one case had been reported in February. All these were considered to be imported outbreaks of small number. Could we have done a more careful investigation? How did the Somalian government view this outbreak?

Finally, after much deliberation and the realisation of the futility of my efforts while in the plane, I decided to get some sleep before I landed.

The airplane landed at Mogadishu airport after skimming over a blue sea and the multi-hued beach of the Indian Ocean. We landed at three o'clock, to the sight of the Somalian national flag (white star on a blue field) flapping in the strong wind. At the airport, waiting for me was the resident WHO Medical Officer, Mahfuz Ali, who greeted me saying, "I haven't seen you for a long time."

Mahfuz Ali and I were reuniting after a long time. Ali used to be a health officer in Pakistan before being employed by the WHO, and was acquainted with me. He informed me that the health minister of Somalia was to depart for China the next afternoon, and he had therefore made an appointment for me to meet him before that.

I asked Ali about the suspected cases. He replied, "three patients are in the quarantine. There are a total of five patients, including two previous patients. I have just received a telegram from Geneva informing that smallpox virus was isolated from the two previous patients." Instantly, my wishful thinking that the positive specimens might be due to vaccinia virus was dashed.

From the airport I directly checked into a hotel called Croce del Sud, run by an Italian. This hotel later became the regular hotel for WHO officers and epidemiologists visiting Somalia. I was put in a large room, surrounded by thick white walls characteristic of south Italy. The hotel had a spacious courtyard with the tables covered by red-check tablecloths. Many Italians still remained in Somalia after independence, running the restaurants and car repair shops, and in trades such as machine tools. At the time, the population of Mogadishu was 400,000, and the town was segregated into two clear parts—a conventional, Italian shopping area, and a region with white clay walls inhabited by the Somalians.

Next morning, at around seven o'clock, I kept my appointment with the health minister. There appeared to be a high degree of tension within the room. I first addressed the minister

> Mr Minister, the sudden occurrence of smallpox in Mogadishu at this time has caused serious concern within WHO. We thought that the occurrence of smallpox cases in Dimo, Ethiopia on August 9 probably was the last case in Africa and the world. So, we must re-examine the situation. WHO will never spare support. The problem is not only for Somalia but also for the entire world.

The minister said,

> Dr Arita, I know well the reason for your immediate visit. But, we don't believe your findings that there are no more smallpox cases occurring in Ethiopia. We think that many cases are still occurring. Unfortunately, Somalia again suffered the damage of smallpox importation from Ethiopia. Thus far Somalia has warned WHO many times of the risk of the outbreak of smallpox in Ethiopia and its consequent spread to Somalia. WHO has not responded to this warning.

Colonel Muse Rabile Goud, the health minister, was a leader of the Somalia Revolutionary Regime. He possessed a bold head, thick eyebrows and piercing eyes, and it was evident that he was a practical man. I responded saying,

> I can understand well what you say. But, the WHO has put the greatest efforts into operations in Ethiopia, both in the Ogaden desert and the highlands. Thousands of Ethiopian programme officers and seven WHO experts are engaged in the search for cases, and containment as needed. All possible transportation means, such as helicopters, cars and camels, were used. The results of this extensive action showed that the last patient was from Dimo. However, we will further reinforce the efforts in Ethiopia. Regarding Somalia, I think that one WHO officer is not enough to support the smallpox eradication work. I would like to have your permission for Dr Anatolij Slepushkin (USSR), my colleague at Geneva, and Dr Stanley Foster of CDC, Atlanta, the United States, to come immediately to Somalia. I would also like to examine the epidemiological situation while visiting your isolation station.

The minister replied, "I agree with the assignment of Dr Slepushkin of WHO, but only one person is enough. I am now leaving for China for a several-week visit from today. I wish that the action will have been completed before I come back".[3]

After my meeting with the health minister, I immediately left for the isolation station with Mahfuz Ali and few Somalian officers. It was located in the eastern part of Mogadishu city. The station turned out to be a house with three rooms and tents, on the premises of the Research Institute of Tuberculosis. Since entry was restricted, the entry gate was locked and a guard stationed to keep watch. We were admitted only after obtaining permission.

The last smallpox patient that I examined was in West Bengal of India in the spring of 1975. Thereafter, smallpox patients had only been found in Ethiopia. As we entered the Research Institute of Tuberculosis I knew that once again I was about to examine four true smallpox patients in Mogadishu.

[3] Author's notes.

13

Mysterious Source of Infection

The first step in any epidemiological investigation is a detailed discussion with the index case or first patient. To obtain the best results it is necessary to establish credibility with the patient. Patients must be convinced of coming to no harm later, even if they speak the truth. At the station, five suspected smallpox patients were registered; of those five, one died.

At first, the Somalian surveillance staff and I sat beside the bed of Faduma Ali Mohammed, one of the four patients (see figure 13.1). She was a woman of about thirty, with a narrow face, slender body and long spindly hands and legs characteristic of Somalis. She had brown skin and refined features, and was wearing a blue scarf on her head and the traditional one-piece cloth with a long train wrapped around her body. Faduma had developed a rash on 17 September. She had never been vaccinated for smallpox. The pustules covering her whole body had just begun to dry.

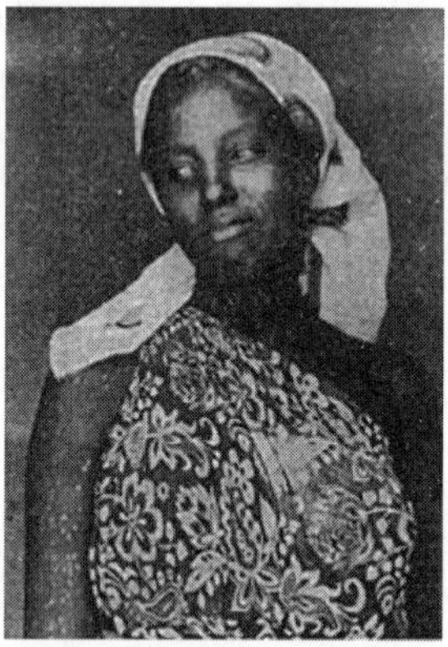

FIGURE 13.1 Patient interviewed in Somalia, 1976

Source: World Health Organization.

I approached Faduma with extreme caution, as I did not wish to scare her.

> I have come from a faraway country. It must have been very painful due to this disease. I am working to get rid of this disease. I have no connection with the army or the police. If you tell me how you got this disease, we can prevent your family and friends from also getting this disease.

In the absence of a response, I continued,

> This disease is called *furuqa* in Somali, as you know. This does not come down from the heaven or emerge from the earth. You got this disease from your friend or acquaintance. You must have surely met a person who suffered from a similar disease previously. Would you tell me where you met such a patient?

I spoke to Faduma with the help of a Somali interpreter who had accompanied me. Faduma was naturally suspicious of strangers. However, before long, she began to talk.

> We are nomads from Mogadishu. We are moving with five family members and fifty-three camels in search of grass and water. How to move? The method for moving is not particularly fixed. We go in the direction where it rains and there is grass. A month ago, we headed to Ramasiling through El Kere (a village of Bale province, Ethiopia). You mean a similar disease? As I recall, at around the place where we were passing El Kere, we met a group of nomads coming from the opposite direction towards us. Yes, we greeted by waving our hands. As I recall, I think that there was a person among them with the disease similar to the one I have. However, we never bivouacked together. When you ask where, I do not know the name of the place. However, the place is about one hour walking distance to the north of El Kere. I remember there were three oases.

Faduma continued to talk. "I have a young sister living in Mogadishu. I come to meet her. I passed Ramasiling and Yet. This rash came out about six days after arriving at Mogadishu. I came by a truck from Yet to Mogadishu."[1]

While listening to Faduma talk, I constructed in my mind a story about the source, date and place of her infection. The date of

[1] Extracts of this conversation from author's notes.

onset of rash of the patient from Dimo, the last known smallpox case in Ethiopia, was 9 August. According to the calculation based on incubation period, the date when Faduma was assumed to be infected after meeting the smallpox patient was around 5 September. However, since the patient from Dimo was completely cured by this time, he could not have been the source of infection for Faduma. It was impossible that Faduma was infected with smallpox by the patient from Dimo. Where, then, was the smallpox patient who had infected Faduma?

It is considered that Faduma had not yet arrived at the frontier town of Yet and, therefore, the infection must have occurred on the Ethiopian side of the border. Did this mean there would be additional smallpox cases in Ethiopia? The last case in Dimo, therefore, was not the last case there? This is a very important point and I strongly felt the need to meet the Ethiopian officers to confirm the story.

After interviewing Faduma, I continued my discussions with the remaining three patients. Finally, two possible sources of infection emerged. One was the region around El Kere, which Faduma referred to, and the other the Kelafo region from where the remaining patients came; all on the Ethiopian side.

On the way back from the quarantine station, I sent a telex from the central post office of Mogadishu to D. A. Henderson in Geneva.

> The five patients in the quarantine, among them one aged seventy years died; four were confirmed clinically to be typical smallpox cases. Regarding infection sources, the region within a 50-kilometre radius centred by El Kere village of Bale province, Ethiopia as well as the region of Kelafo and the village of El Abred is suspicious. Please make arrangements for me to meet the WHO smallpox group of Ethiopia at Ferfer or Yet situated along the Ethiopia and Somalia border. [2]

Ferfer is a village at the border of Somalia and Ethiopia, located at the end of the main road, 350 kilometres north of Mogadishu. At the time, it was a small village with roughly twenty houses. The "houses" were actually small crude huts with roofs of shrub branches from the desert and walls made of dry weed, sufficient to

[2] Author's notes.

provide shade and some relief from the hot sun. Across 300 metres of no-man's land, the roof of the border patrol building of Ethiopia could be seen. The programme officers from Somalia and Ethiopia could finally meet at Ferfer.

On 3 October 1976, Mahfuz Ali, members of the Somalian group and I walked through no-man's land in the hot sun, following the instructions of the Ethiopian border patrol. Ali cautioned the Somalian group, "Don't get excited. Talk quietly." After walking about 100 metres, we saw the Ethiopian group walking towards us from the Ethiopian station. I saw a few WHO officers: Bert van Ramshorst (the Netherlands) who covered the Kelafo region, Jean Paul Ryst (France) who covered the Gode region, and Carl Hasselblad (United States) and Mohamed El Naggar (Egypt) who covered the El Kere region. I heard that the first three men had arrived by road in a Toyota Land Cruiser and El Naggar by air in a WHO helicopter. All the men were in their thirties, and were engaged in the search for smallpox cases in the Ogaden desert on the Ethiopian side. Van Ramshorst wore a khaki shirt and sunglasses. Ryst had on a shabby shirt, an oddly shaped hat and sandals, and Hasselblad whose face was covered with a beard, wore a military uniform. El Naggar wore a neat, open grey shirt. In fact, these men were to be part of the WHO global smallpox eradication programme right till the end, having devoted themselves during the most difficult time of the campaign. We laughed together on meeting again, unexpectedly, in this most unlikely place.

Van Ramshorst asked, "By the way, what did the smallpox patients in Mogadishu say about the source of the infection?" I explained in detail. "The region within a 50-kilometre radius centred by El Kere is most suspicious. Especially, the region near El Kere with the three oases is most suspicious. Carl, according to your report no smallpox case has been found in this region for the last four months. Is it sure?" Hasselblad replied,

> I have continued to walk for the last four months from nomad to nomad, and from settlement to settlement searching for cases. Since 9 August when the patient of Dimo was found, no new smallpox case has been found. According to my policy, I do not use a helicopter. If I fly in the air, I would miss cases. However, I might have missed the cases. I understand

well. I will examine once more. It will take another four months, but even so I must do it.[3]

These words of Hasselblad represent the attitude of our WHO officers at the time while the search for smallpox was on. In fact, true to his word, Hasselblad combed the entire problem region again for six months. Although the three oases that Faduma had mentioned were found, even one smallpox case was not found. Till today we do not know whether (a) Faduma's understanding was at fault; (b) Faduma had lied; (c) the interpreter had mistranslated what Faduma had said; or, (d) if smallpox cases had been missed in El Kere. The mode of smallpox transmission indicates that the presence of a patient surely means the existence of another patient as the source. Taking into consideration the fact that it was unlikely that smallpox cases would not be recognised despite a patient and meticulous search, I believe even now that the source of infection was not in the region within a 50-kilometre radius in El Kere.

New Smallpox Report from Kenya

In December 1976, in Nairobi, the Virus Research Institute reported on the results of the analysis of a specimen taken from a suspected smallpox case found in Mandera province, northern Kenya. At that time, as the global programme stood on the threshold of success, it was the practice that every suspected case of smallpox (even if there was only the slightest doubt that it was smallpox) had to be subject to laboratory investigation. This practice was only started in 1973 and was continued until the end of the programme. Prior to this, WHO had recommended that it was more practical in the countries endemic for smallpox to diagnose smallpox based on clinical manifestations of the disease. In retrospect, this was the correct method of smallpox surveillance.

In the laboratory test, the sample was inoculated into eggs, which were kept at 37° C for three days. The eggs were opened after three days to find the result. The virologist at the Nairobi Virus Research Institute was puzzled by some unexpected findings.

[3] Extract of conversation between the three men from author's notes.

There were whitish lesions of 1–2 millimetres in diameter on the surface of a special membrane in the egg. Such lesions suggested that the specimens might contain smallpox virus or herpes virus. However, the last smallpox case in Kenya was in 1974, with two years having passed without any cases. The report of the last smallpox case in Ethiopia was in August 1976. This was unlikely to have any correlation with the present occurrence. In Somalia, the adjacent country, ongoing smallpox outbreaks were reported in the capital Mogadishu, but this was situated more than 500 kilometres from Mandera. Despite the doubts that the specimen was really smallpox, the aliquot of the specimen was urgently sent through the WHO smallpox office in Geneva to the WHO Smallpox Reference Laboratory, CDC, in Atlanta. The reference laboratory isolated the smallpox virus from the specimen five days later.

How the smallpox infection was transmitted to Mandera was a mystery which puzzled all of us. What was going on in the Horn of Africa? WHO had to investigate, to provide the answers. Finally, the entire story did come to light.

Walking around the desert regions of Somalia, one sometimes comes across a small Koranic school. Under a big tree, forty to fifty small children between the ages of five to ten sit and learn. A slim white-haired old man in a white robe is usually the teacher and he teaches the Koran to the children. The sentences of the Koran, printed onto a wooden plate, serve as the textbook of this open-air classroom. Hassan was a travelling teacher of such a Koranic school. It was around 25 December 1976 when he visited a small village, Ledi, of Mandera province, Kenya, after crossing the border from Somalia. He stayed at the house where his mother lived. I heard that during this time Hassan had developed a rash and fever. It was Hassan who turned out to be the cause of the four smallpox cases of this family. The last patient was a four-month old girl, and the date of the onset of her rash was recorded to be 2 February 1977, the last smallpox case in Kenya.

However, the problem was to find the source of infection. Undeniably, the cases in Kenya were caused by Hassan, a patient from outside of Kenya. But one big question remained unanswered, where was Hassan infected from?

Undoubtedly, Hassan must have had contact with some smallpox outbreak that had occurred during that period. Without the least delay, after receiving confirmation that the Mandera cases were smallpox, instructions via telegram from Geneva were sent to the smallpox operations centre in Mogadishu.

> The Koran teacher, Hassan, is considered to be the source of the smallpox outbreak in Kenya. Contact all the Koran schools in the city of Mogadishu, and ask whether the Koran teacher, Hassan, is known or not. If he is known, examine in detail his activity for the last two months and report it. In addition, also regarding the smallpox patients in Mogadishu found in November, examine whether Hassan had contact with the patients.[4]

Investigations in Mogadishu led to two persons named Hassan being found, but they were different from the Koran teacher in question. There was no trace of the Hassan who was the source of the Mandera cases anywhere in Mogadishu.

Investigators did uncover a relative of the Koran teacher Hassan, at a place near a sugar factory in Jowhar town, about 80 kilometres north of Mogadishu. Subsequently, this place was also examined but the search proved inconclusive. Instructions were also sent to El Kere, in the region of the Ogaden desert in Ethiopia, since the last outbreak occurred there in August 1976. Again, the answer was in the negative; a Koran teacher by the name of Hassan was not known.

As mentioned earlier, if one smallpox case is found, another smallpox case should certainly have existed somewhere, two to three weeks prior to the second case. The location and date of the smallpox occurrences around Somalia known at that time are shown in table 13.1.

TABLE 13.1 Last smallpox case in Ethiopia, Somalia and Kenya

Location	*Date*
Dimo village, El Kere, Ethiopia	9 August 1976
Mogadishu city, Somalia	from September 1976 to January 1977
Ledi, Mandera, Kenya	5 February 1977

[4] Author's notes.

Transmission of smallpox virus in Ethiopia was ended on 9 August 1976. The cases in Mogadishu occurred one month after the cases in Dimo village of Ethiopia, but the correlation between them is not known, as already mentioned. Therefore, some smallpox cases that the WHO did not know of occurred in the triangle shaped region between these three places. That is, the hidden foci of smallpox might have been somewhere in this triangle region (see map 13.1).

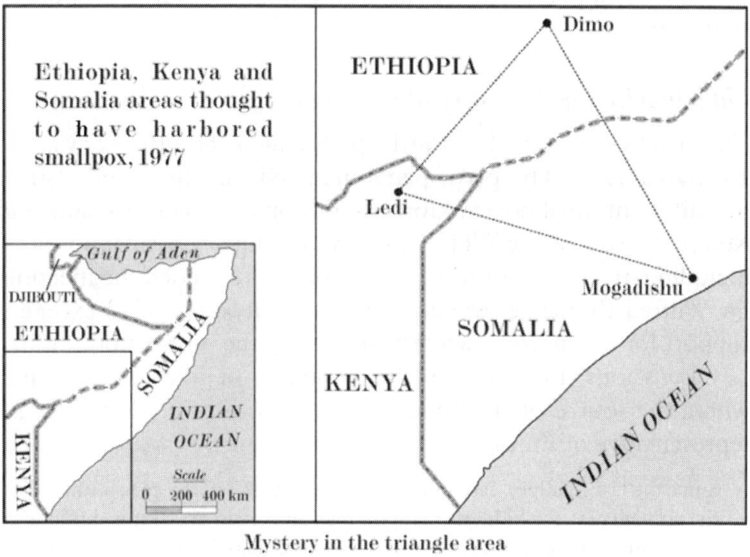

Map 13.1 Mystery in the Triangle Area

Source: World Health Organization.

At the time, the region within this triangle was part of the three-way conflict zone between the governments of Somalia, Ethiopia and Kenya. This has been discussed in detail in chapter 12. Guerrilla activity within this zone of conflict complicated any smallpox search operations. Thus, owing to the circumstances in the Ogaden desert, the border region between the three countries was politically unstable, which presented great obstacles for WHO to handle the end game of smallpox eradication.

How was WHO to proceed? We felt the solution might lie in open communication and information exchange between officers of the three countries in question—Somalia, Ethiopia and Kenya.

This proposal of WHO, to hold such a meeting, was readily accepted by the three nations. It was decided that the meeting would be held in Nairobi, the capital of Kenya, in March 1977. Sudan, as Ethiopia's neighbour, also attended. Sudan recorded its last smallpox case in 1973, but still continued countermeasures from the standpoint that the risk of importation from Ethiopia was significant.

Nairobi Meeting: "Mystery in the Triangle Area"

The meeting was held at the Department of Health, Kenya, 14–16 March 1977. The participants included the chiefs and staff of the different smallpox taskforces—Ethiopia, Sudan, Somalia and Kenya—as well as the WHO local and headquarters smallpox staff, including me. A total of nearly thirty officers attended the meeting. Dr Wilfred Koinange, Medical Officer, Kenya, provided excellent support for the meeting while representing the host nation.

Discussions focused on the problem of the triangle area where the source of smallpox infection was possibly hidden. The representative of Ethiopia stated:

> Since the last smallpox case in Dimo in August 1976, Ethiopia continued the surveillance for hidden smallpox foci. In certain areas, it is difficult due to guerrilla activities. Nevertheless, more than 200 specimens were collected from smallpox suspects. The laboratory studies revealed all of them as negative for smallpox.

This is what the representative of Kenya said.

> In the Mandera district, the smallpox importation was discovered and we completely examined this district. The problem is that 80 per cent of the population in this district is nomadic, and they have no borders. From Sidamo or Bale Provinces, Ethiopia, or from southern Somalia, nomads visit our country to seek water and grass, and then leave at any time. Nobody can control their movements. However, the examination thus far indicates that smallpox was imported by a Somali named Hassan, and we can affirm that there are no secondary cases in Mandera district. The main point is to confirm quickly that there is no smallpox in the

surrounding area other than Mandera. I think that joint surveillance efforts are needed in the border areas.

Somalia's stand on the issue was as follows.

We made our best effort to examine the source of smallpox infection in Kenya, the teacher Hassan. Unfortunately, we could not obtain any useful information. Hassan possibly did not return to Somalia after his visit to Mandera. Then, where is he? It's hard to say. The smallpox outbreaks in Mogadishu are being gotten under control. No secondary cases have been found since January 17.

The Sudanese representative commented on the talks:

Ethiopia, Kenya and Somalia insist that there is no smallpox case in its territory, but then from where did the source of smallpox infection in Kenya come from? At present, the only place in the world that smallpox is occurring is in this region of the Horn of Africa. The fact that the infection source of Kenya has not been elucidated means that smallpox is occurring somewhere in this region of the Horn of Africa. Unless smallpox disappears from this region, and unless this fact is verified, it cannot be said that the world is freed from smallpox. The answer is only one, the strengthening of smallpox surveillance in the Horn of Africa, with main emphasis on the triangle area, that's it. Our country Sudan is far from the mysterious triangle area, but we will enforce further the surveillance. I wish that Kenya, Ethiopia and Somalia also reinforce further the smallpox surveillance. We should then certainly find the foci. The method is well known according the experience in the eradication program of the past 10 years. There's no smoke without fire.[5]

This statement from Sudan was well accepted by the individual national representatives. Notably, the participating nations decided to make unified efforts for the success of the smallpox eradication programme in the Horn of Africa, regardless of their own political standpoint on the Ogaden desert.

The meeting was adjourned after having pledged that (a) under the coordination of WHO, the three nations would intensify surveillance with exchange of information, and (b) another coordination meeting would be held in Nairobi after six months, in September 1977, to re-examine the situation.

[5] Arita, *Smallpox Eradication*; Fenner et al., *Smallpox and its Eradication*.

14

Emergency Countermeasures Against the Smallpox Epidemic in Somalia

Ehsan Shafa, an Iranian member of the WHO smallpox team in Geneva, and the Somali smallpox chief flew together to Mogadishu immediately after the Nairobi meeting. As described previously, Shafa was my colleague since the start of the programme in 1967 and was respected in African and Asian countries where the smallpox eradication programme was underway because of his good and friendly character and active work style.

As soon as Shafa landed at the Mogadishu airport, the Somali team received the following information: "A smallpox-like case occurred in Fuda village, Bakool region."

This was the first case in Somalia that was reported from a region other than the capital, Mogadishu. Ironically, Fuda (about 250 kilometres away, northwest from Mogadishu) is in a region located almost at the centre of the mysterious triangular point, situated along the road connecting Ethiopia, Ogaden and Somalia, used frequently by nomads. Shafa immediately rushed to Fuda village with a Somali team. The patient was confirmed as a case of smallpox. Investigation of the report of this outbreak gradually revealed that the regions in southern Somalia had been heavily infected with smallpox outbreaks and that epidemics were continuing. The transmission initially occurred along the main road, from Mogadishu to Baidoa, and then began to spread to nomad areas away from the road. Outbreak investigations further revealed the epidemiological features of the disease.

First, symptoms were mild, resembling the mild smallpox occurring in southern Ethiopia, Brazil, Botswana and elsewhere. The mortality rate was only about 1 per cent. This particular strain could be classified as variola minor or variola intermediate type, although the initial symptoms at the onset of rash are indistinguishable from those of severe Asian-type smallpox (variola major). Second, nomads usually wander as a group of forty people, within a desert area of roughly 200 kilometres, to seek water and grass. The transmission of the smallpox virus, it was found, among such groups, could sustain for as long as 207 days.

The vaccination coverage was high (about 70 per cent) in the villages along the main roads, but very low (less than 10 per cent) among the nomads found about 15 kilometres from the road. These were the reasons why smallpox transmission was sustained in the Ogaden. And the smallpox importation from the Ethiopian side of the Ogaden to Somalia through nomad movements could be easily suspected. The investigation results caused concern about the further spread of smallpox to Kenya or Djibouti.

Experience urged further, broader action, in addition to containment of the epidemics in Somalia. The principal concern was the impending Muslim pilgrimage to Mecca in November. What would happen if a pilgrim from Somalia transported the smallpox virus into Mecca? Just the thought was terrifying. In Mecca, a total of 2 million from more than fifty nations were anticipated to gather. The implication of the smallpox virus being transmitted among such a large and heterogeneous number was alarming. Put simply, it meant smallpox spreading to the various countries of Asia and Africa once the Muslim pilgrims returned to their respective countries.

Finally, there was a question mark on Somalia's capability in terms of capacity and resources to control the spread of smallpox within its borders. The last, large outbreak of smallpox in Somalia had been in the early 1960s. Since then, Somalia had no experience in controlling the disease on a large scale.

Thus, several grave problems were anticipated at the time. I describe here the situation on the ground in terms of the success or failure of WHO's actions, which in turn directly impacted the failure/success of the smallpox eradication programme.

At first, an emergency message was sent from the WHO Geneva Smallpox Unit to the WHO Regional Office for South-East Asia in New Delhi: "In view of the urgency to contain the smallpox epidemics in Somalia, would appreciate your dispatching three to four WHO smallpox field workers from Indian programme to Mogadishu soonest." [1]

At this point, India was about to complete the two-year term for searching for smallpox cases. The response was rapid. The regional office dispatched four WHO smallpox field staff to Mogadishu within two months, having rearranged their tight schedule in their own Indian field operations. One of the people assigned was Rodney Hatfield (from UK), the member of the operations team, who managed several hundred cars for the eradication programme in Bihar and was also responsible for the management of the finances of the programme. On arrival, he took the post of the head of the management of the smallpox office for the Somalia programme. Zdeno Jezek (from Czechoslovakia) was the head of the WHO smallpox eradication team in India (as has been mentioned in chapter 8). In Somalia, accurate epidemiological assessment of the smallpox situation was urgently required to develop the most effective measures for interruption of transmission. Jezek already had extensive experience with this kind of work during his few years working for the programme. He became the chief of the WHO smallpox fieldwork in Mogadishu to manage the global end game in Somalia. Mohamed Al Aghbari (from Yemen) had covered several states near New Delhi, and was once the Minister of Health, Yemen. He was familiar with handling collaboration among Islamic nations. In addition to the field operations, he was made in-charge of communications and relations with the government as a WHO spokesman.

Remarkably, as soon as the smallpox outbreak in Somalia was known to the world community, I received numerous letters from friends, colleagues and even those whom I had never met but who had worked with the smallpox eradication programme in Asia, the Americas, Africa and Europe. The following words sum up the content of their messages. "I learned of the outbreak in the press. I worry very much about the matter. Please tell me without hesitation,

[1] Author's notes.

if I can do anything to help. Field work in Somalia may be difficult, so I heard, but I am ready to start working any time."[2]

In late May Somalia prepared for action. Abdullahi Deria was assigned as the national programme manager. Coincidentally, Shafa had happened to meet Deria while travelling from London to Mogadishu and had talked with Deria about the smallpox programme.[3] This discussion led to Deria becoming interested in the programme. Subsequently, we (on the WHO side) welcomed Deria's offer of help towards the national programme. It was our good fortune that we got the correct person at the correct time in this crucial and difficult situation. Deria, as the chief, was assisted by twenty Somalian programme staff and by fifteen WHO staff members. Since his joining, Deria and I often worked together.

We had a further run of good luck when Bert Van Ramshorst, Carl Hasselblad, Mohamed El Naggar and Jean Paul Ryst also joined the team. As mentioned in an earlier chapter, I had met them in 1976 at Ferfer at the Somalia-Ethiopia border, and all of them were specialists of the Ogaden Desert Program. Stanley Foster, who once was the WHO chief of the Bangladesh smallpox eradication programme, also joined in from the US. Parenthetically, there were many other officers who worked for this special operation effectively. Regrettably I am not able to mention all of them.

As soon as Jezek arrived, he was absorbed in the preparation of the plan for the operation. Although active case search, containment operations and the strategy remained the same, he struggled to determine what would work best in the specific environment of desert and nomads. The points of the plan are listed here.

1. Respect the priorities. Apply maximal manpower into the regions with the highest reported incidence, putting off the regions with low incidence.
2. Employ workers directly from nomad persons who have basic reading and writing skills, and carry out the search for hidden cases, to the maximum extent, by using these persons.

[2] Author's notes.

[3] Deria was returning to Somalia after completing his studies at the London School of Hygiene and Tropical Medicine.

3. Provide reward money; 200 Somali schillings (about US $30), to a person who reports a new smallpox case.

Essential paperwork and materials to be carried by workers was prepared, and Jezek provided necessary briefing to the WHO short-term staff arriving in the country, and sent them to the areas where the outbreaks were heaviest.

As for the vaccine, the stock-piled vaccine of Geneva was used. However, there remained one large problem, namely, a shortage of transport. At least sixteen vehicles were required, immediately.

The Land Rover, produced by Leyland Motors (UK), was a car suitable for fieldwork. However, it took a minimum of twelve months from order to on-site receipt. This was too long a wait for the eradication programme staff. At the beginning of the year, in February and March, few Land Rover/Toyota vehicles had been purchased on-site in Nairobi and sent by ground transportation from there to Mogadishu. However, this method was inadequate in meeting the minimum transportation needs of the team.

In mid May 1977, John Wickett (from Canada), the administrative officer of the WHO Smallpox Eradication Unit, Ron Hauge (from the US), the supply officer of the unit, and myself were struggling to solve the problem of shortage of transport. We discussed the problem at length and the possible solutions:

> Sixteen more Land Rovers are needed. Now, we are using 34 cars that are fully occupied by the staff to control the outbreaks in south Somalia. In Somalia, there are 16 regions, each of which need one car at least; a total of 16 cars are by any means necessary. The surveillance needs to be intensified in every region, otherwise we will fail to finish this end game. This is based on the plan that the smallpox outbreaks can be contained and assuming no transmission in the other regions. At worst, the outbreak spreads to the other regions. How to handle, then? It may be hard to use the current 34 cars already assigned to the outbreak control in the south. In any case, 16 cars are the minimum requirement.
>
> Sixteen cars at US $10,000 each means that a total of US $160,000 is necessary. Do we have the money? Furthermore, if we need them urgently, we have no choice other than air transport, and then does WHO have the experience of air transportation? If they are sent by air, an additional US $10,000 for air freight may be necessary for each car.

> We can still pay the money from the funds donated last year. However, since the course of the outbreak of Somalia cannot be predicted, a cost of as much as US $320,000 including the cost of air transport is a big risk. If the outbreak expands, we have no money left at all. [4]

Hauge interrupted the conversation:

> I just called Copenhagen. I learned that we can buy at least 16 Land Rovers right now. That is, if we make a contract now. I asked the other capitals of Europe, but the 16 cars from Copenhagen are the most promising. Anyway, we need 16 cars, don't we? It is a well paying gamble if the cars are immediately sent by air transport to Somalia at a cost of US $320,000 and the outbreak can be controlled, even though it may be a big risk.

To this Wickett replied, "There is the Coordinator's office of the United Nations Disaster Relief Organization (UNDRO) in Geneva. If Somalia asks for aid from this office by designating the smallpox outbreak as a national disaster emergency, special funding may possibly be obtained from UNDRO."

"Does UNDRO have contingency funds?" asked Hauge.

"No", replied Wickett, "when they receive the request for aid for a disaster emergency, they appeal to national governments via telegram. They have a strategy to get the acceptance of the national governments."

"I understand, we need to take UNDRO into consideration. I will inform it to Somalia right now", said Hauge. [5]

We eventually arrived at the following conclusions:

1. A total of sixteen cars needed to be sent by air transport.
2. For this purpose, we would purchase the Land Rovers from Europe, using the money at hand.
3. Simultaneously, we would try and raise funds by appealing to UNDRO. If we could raise the funds through UNDRO, it would be OK. If we couldn't, we would face financial difficulty soon. However, with no choice in the matter, we had to do what we could without further delay.

[4] Conversation between author and Wickett. From author's notes.

[5] From author's notes.

4. Our immediate costs were roughly US $400,000. This would cover the purchase of sixteen Land Rovers, with necessary spare parts and tires, and also the cost of sending them to Somalia by air transport.

Busy days began in Geneva. On 18 May 1977, the Government of Somalia sent a telegram to UNDRO, through WHO.

> The big outbreak of smallpox is bringing about a serious threat to Somalia and to the global smallpox eradication program. The severity of the outbreak and its circumstances cannot be controlled by the resources available in Somalia. We are asking the following aid as soon as possible: air transportation of 16 Land Rovers with spare parts, tires and the like.[6]

UNDRO on its part required a confirmation vis-à-vis the telegram from the United Nations office in Mogadishu. First, did the chief of the UN office in Mogadishu consider this appeal to be justifiable? Second, as Somalia at the time was one of the most highly armed countries in the Horn of Africa, was it possible that it could receive this aid from the army?

The Mogadishu office confirmed the justifiability of the telegram from Somalia, and said that the aid from the army was out of the question due to the political climate of the region.

On May 27, UNDRO accepted the request from Somalia and dispatched the telegram to the listed nations for donation of transport and other supplies to Somalia so that their existing smallpox epidemics may be controlled. The responses of the donor nations to this request were immediate (see table 14.1).

The sixteen vehicles were finally obtained. A number of the Land Rovers in Copenhagen were reserved for use in emergencies by UNICEF, but twelve of these were diverted to WHO. Another three cars were provided by the UK from stocks already planned for other aid programmes; and the International Red Cross provided the last one.

[6] Arita, *Smallpox Eradication*.

TABLE 14.1 Money donated by donor nations, 30 May–30 June 1977

Date of Offer	*Donor*	*Amount of Money (US$)*
30 May 1977	United Kingdom	74,000
1 June 1977	Norway	9,500
1 June 1977	The Netherlands	65,000
1 June 1977	IFRC*	42,000
3 June 1977	Canada	100,000
3 June 1977	Sweden	120,000
30 June 1977	Sweden (again)	50,000
		465,000

Note: *International Federation of Red Cross and Red Crescent Societies.

Transporting the sixteen Land Rovers by air proved complicated. It required considerable paperwork and procedures such as selection of a company for the airlift, date of supply, permission for air travel and landing, etc., needed to be sorted out. All these details had to be finalised in consultation with the nations involved in the flight schedule of the airplane that was transporting the vehicles. Finally, after much effort, all the details were worked out and arrangements made to begin transporting the cars (See figure 14.1).

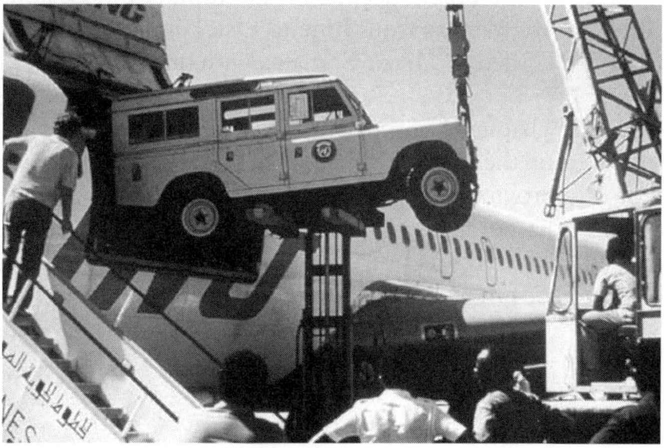

FIGURE 14.1 Vehicles being airlifted into Somalia for the 1977 emergency

Source: World Health Organization.

The first four cars departed on 3 June from Manston airport, UK, in a Stretch Hercules (C130) airplane, that arrived in Mogadishu the next day. The next three cars departed on 3 June from Copenhagen, but due to office procedures in Athens were delayed and arrived in Mogadishu only on 8 June. The third air transport consignment of three cars departed as on 7 June, and arrived at Mogadishu on 9 June. The forth air consignment, with the remaining six cars, departed Copenhagen on 13 June and arrived in Mogadishu on 14 June.

Spare parts, tyres and other materials such as vaccine and posters necessary for the Somalia programme were collected in Copenhagen, and were simultaneously loaded onto the aircraft with the vehicles. Twenty-five days had gone by since the telegram from Somalia on 18 May requesting emergency aid. While the air transportation of the vehicles was underway, the Somali outbreak response activities improved rapidly. Twenty-three WHO staff and consultants were engaged in the response effort, along with 3,000 local health workers mobilised by the Somali government. The total number of vehicles for the programme reached fifty, which met the immediate needs.

After the initial phase of the emergency response, which had been haphazard and disorganised, the containment activities made rapid progress, with a rapid decline in the number of cases during the following five months from June to October 1977. Finally, the last case was recorded in Merca, Somalia, with onset on 26 October 1977.

In the next chapter, I will discuss in detail the response in the Ogaden desert on the Ethiopian side of the border even as the Somali operation was proving to be increasingly effective. For us, work on both sides of the border was essential to the eradication effort for the area being covered was really one single epidemiological area in which the nomads moved freely across the border frontiers.

15

End Game in Ethiopia, Again: Was it Really Smallpox Free?

The reports of the smallpox outbreaks in Somalia were well known to Kenya, Ethiopia and Djibouti thorough the WHO communication channels (see maps 15.1 and 15.2). All these countries had issued warnings about the risk of importations and had reinforced their search for smallpox cases. Ethiopia presented special difficulties. In 1977, in the three provinces that included Ogaden desert areas—Bale, Sidamo and Hararge—the guerrilla activities of the Western Somalia Liberation Front (which had the objective of gaining independence from Ethiopia) had increased substantially, which made the implementation and execution of the smallpox eradication programme very difficult.

On 1 June 1977, I flew in a small airplane from Addis Ababa to Gode, a critical centre of the programme in the Ogaden desert. The national project manager, Ato Yemane, and his WHO counterpart, Mahendra Dutta, were with me. The guerrilla activity of the Western Somalia Liberation Front appeared to be at its peak. No security staff of the United Nations was present, as all had been pulled back. Only the WHO smallpox programme officers remained because the Ogaden smallpox project was accorded the highest priority in the global eradication programme. However, we were concerned about the risks of continuing the programme, especially if the operations were life threatening to the staff. The main purpose of my visit was to see whether or not the staff should stay and continue the work given the regular guerrilla activities.

The airplane threaded through the clouds to turn south-east over the central mountainous areas of Ethiopia, and changed direction at Bildaw to fly south-west straight to Gode. Within ten minutes from Bildaw we entered the dry land of the Ogaden desert. From the airplane I could see the crossing red lines, like a plaid design, remnants of oil-searching companies from North America that had made vertical and horizontal markings to show the areas investigated.

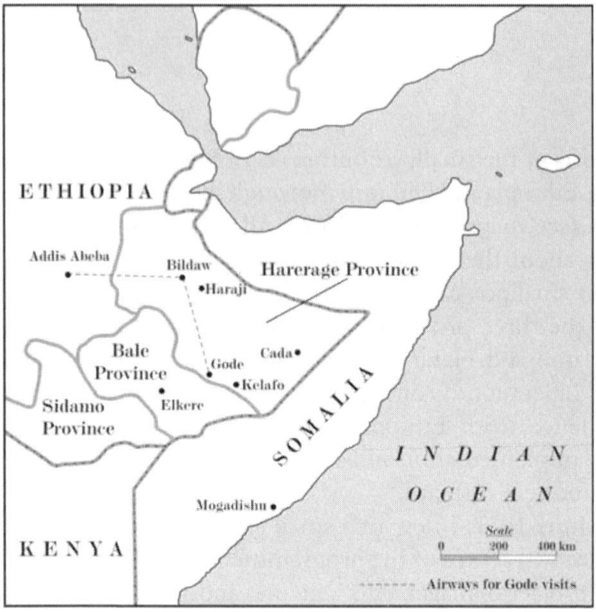

MAP 15.1 Situation of Ogaden Desert and Ethiopia

Source: World Health Organization.

In Gode, the WHO team was being engaged in active search for smallpox cases. The small Gode airport had only one airstrip. Alex Gromyko (from USSR), a member of the WHO smallpox team from Geneva, met us at the airstrip holding his hair against the strong wind. In addition to Gromyko, there were a few staff members too: Poerwokoesoemo Arbani (from Indonesia) who worked in Kelafo, Claudio Amaral (from Brazil) who worked in Warder, and El Naggar (from Egypt) who worked in El Kere. All of these areas fell within the mysterious triangle area (mentioned in chapter 13). We went directly from the airport to the Gode project office, which consisted of barracks.

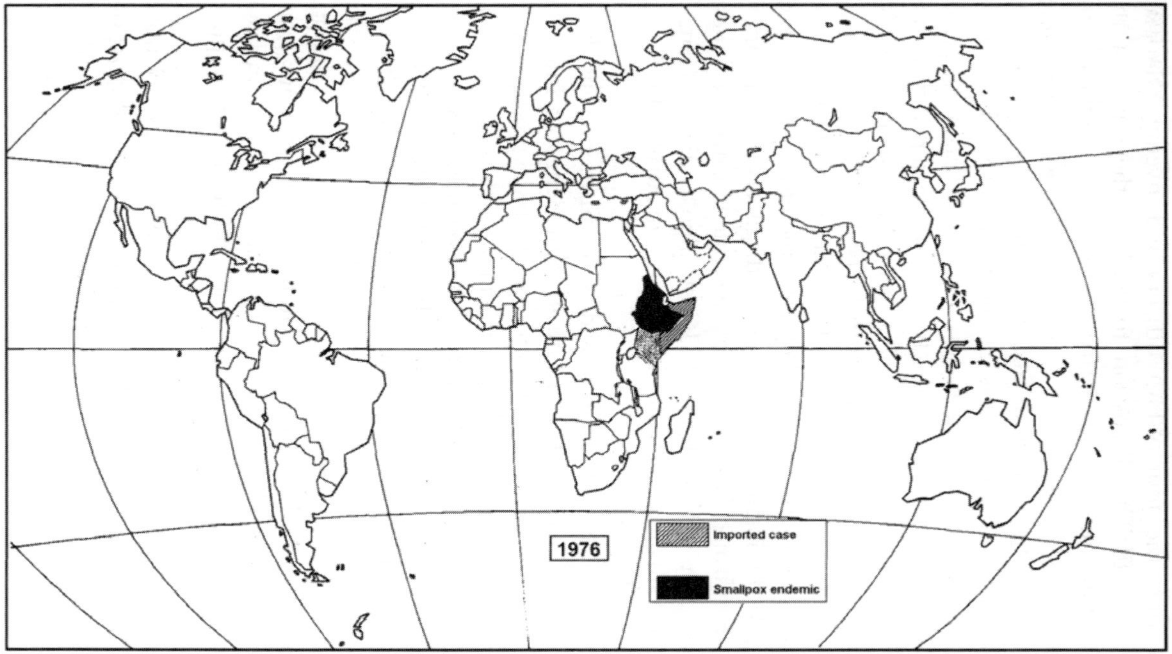

Map 15.2 1976, Smallpox endemic countries and those with importations, 1976.

Source: World Health Organization.

At the meeting place, I discussed the smallpox and security situation with the four WHO officers and twenty Ethiopian programme staff. The discussion focused on the status of the searches and the number of reported suspected cases in the region, which so far, after examination, luckily had left no cases strongly suspected as smallpox. After our talk, we began to review the security problems. Free movement was becoming increasingly difficult due to guerrilla activity in the regions outside the main villages of Kelafo, Warder, El Kere and Gode. It was confirmed that there was no way to maintain effective surveillance except by augmenting the team members by recruiting new Somali-speaking local workers. It was these indigenous people whom the Western Somalia Liberation Front was trying to liberate and they were therefore relatively safe compared to the highland Ethiopians. A diagnosis on a specimen could be confirmed by sending the specimens carried by these indigenous people through the WHO smallpox office in Geneva to the WHO smallpox reference laboratories in Atlanta, USA, and Moscow, USSR.

At this point, I would like to provide some further details about Claudio Amaral. I worked with him in West Bengal in India for three months during the intensive phase of the India programme in the mid-1970s. In the West Bengal programme, the state smallpox eradication office was in Calcutta (now Kolkata). I became the temporary chief of the office from the WHO side, supervising thirteen operational teams, with each assigned to specific districts. Every two months, all the teams returned to Calcutta for a state meeting. It was interesting to remember that whenever, at the end of the meeting, I asked Amaral "Claudio, when will your team depart from Calcutta?" his response was always, "Well, an hour later." Amaral gave this reply every time, and it, in fact, inspired other teams.

Now in Gode, Amaral said, "The region of my charge, Warder, is the safest place among these four regions. I have another report of a smallpox outbreak to be investigated quickly. When I return to Warder tomorrow, I will start immediately on the investigation."[1]

[1] Author's notes.

After the meeting at Gode, I flew again to Bildaw the same day, staying overnight, and arrived at Addis Ababa the next day. At Bildaw I had dinner with a Swedish pilot named Von Rosen. He was about sixty years old. He helped the programme a great deal by flying the smallpox staff in the Horn of Africa. On arrival at Addis Ababa, I reported to the UN safety control officer at the offices of the Economic Commission for Africa of the United Nations. I told him that the WHO Ogaden smallpox eradication programme would continue for a while. After my report, I flew back to Geneva.

The optimistic scenario given by the WHO staff in Gode was not to be matched by the unfortunate events that followed. I soon received information that Claudio Amaral had been captured by guerrillas in the Ogaden. In the following extract, Dr Amaral describes the events around his kidnapping, in his own words.

> At 7 o'clock in the morning of June 3, I started with my Somali colleagues from Warder by car. The destination was the village of Arabra, a small settlement 120 kilometers north from Warder. According to an urgent report, there is a smallpox outbreak there that we must examine without delay.
>
> The sky of the Ogaden desert was blue and everything seemed to go right. However, after we had travelled 80 kilometers, suddenly two men came at us firing machine guns at random and ordered us to stop.
>
> Within three to four minutes, more than a dozen men came out from bushes and surrounded our car. A man came up, and ordered us to leave the car and lie down on the ground, threatening us with a machine gun. A body check was done, and all our belongings were taken away. I wondered if this would be my last day. However, the leader suddenly appeared and ordered us to get in the car again. One of them drove the car and we arrived at a small settlement about 300 meters away. There we were placed in a camp.
>
> I wore shorts because it was hot, but I was ordered to wear Somali clothes. I explained that I was a staff member of the WHO smallpox eradication programme and how smallpox is a dreadful infectious disease. However, the leader said that you cannot work in this region and ordered us to stay with them until it was decided what to do with us. Camel milk was provided as food. Our car was hidden by covering it with tree branches. We were escorted by a man with a machine gun. They were from the Western Somalia Liberation Front.

In the morning of the next day, the leader went out somewhere driving in our car. At about 4 o'clock in the evening, we heard a roar. The helicopter of the smallpox eradication programme was coming to look for us. The guerrilla members became tense and decided on the procedure to capture the helicopter when it landed. We hid as soon as possible. That is because if the helicopter found us it would land to rescue us. When it landed, it would be captured. Fortunately, the helicopter continued on to Warder. We slept again in the camp that night.

In the morning of June 5, we heard again the roar. It was the roar of the same helicopter as yesterday. The guerrilla leader ordered me to communicate by radio to the pilot to land. I lied that I cannot communicate by my portable radio. Then, the leader ordered me to be naked to the waist so that the white skin contrasted well with the brown ground to attract the attention of the pilot. I said that the helicopter was too high to attract such an attention, and I hid myself under a tree. The helicopter flew away again to Warder.

I was fortunate because under such a situation the guerrilla leader began to hear my talk about the smallpox eradication programme, and called the health staff of Arabra village. The health staff reported that the patient of his village [had] chickenpox and not smallpox. Therefore, we attained the aim of the search, although by an odd method. At the night of the same day, we were moved to a neighboring village.

In the morning of June 6, I had a chance to take a walk with the leader together with a security guard, and I talk again earnestly about the smallpox eradication control programme and WHO. I must make them understand the programme by using a chance like this. Finally, the guerrilla leader seemed to believe our status. [2]

Thereafter, the team members, including Amaral, were set free by the guerrillas. They entered into Somalia by crossing the border and eventually returned from Mogadishu to Addis Ababa using a flight arranged by WHO.

I think there were two factors responsible for saving Amaral's life. First, his cool detachment and his enthusiasm for the smallpox eradication programme, which impressed the guerrilla leader. Second, the fact that the guerrilla members always carefully listened to the radio broadcasts from Ethiopia and Somalia, and to the BBC

[2] Report of Claudio Amaral Jr, WHO Epidemiologist Addis Ababa, 25 June 1977.

broadcasts, and were therefore somewhat in touch with the smallpox eradication programme of WHO which was often mentioned in broadcasts. There is also another possibility. When I spoke to the Minister of Health in Somalia about the incident, it is possible that he immediately took action and contacted the office of the Western Somalia Liberation Front about releasing Amaral and his team.

However, the situation in Ogaden was already becoming very tense. Bert van Ramshorst was also captured by guerrillas in the Kelafo region, but subsequently was safely released. He had also discussed the WHO smallpox programme with his captors. El Naggar in El Kere region often encountered guerrillas on his way to investigate cases, and only his wit and his devotion to Islam saved him.

One time, when El Naggar met a guerrilla in a village, he was able to continue his trip in the desert simply saying: "The Koran's teachings are to be faithful to one's duty. I will faithfully carry out smallpox eradication. You do the duty that you believe. However, to interfere is against the Koran's teachings."

However, there was one tragic fatality among the international staff working on smallpox eradication in the Ogaden that shocked us all. The Swedish pilot, Von Rosen, was providing valuable help to the programme by flying smallpox staff and supplies. Tragically, while on duty, he was killed during an attack by guerrillas in Gode, shocking and saddening us all.

The Ogaden Desert Becomes a Battlefield

Finally, in July 1977, the Somali army swept through the Ogaden desert—including Kelafo, Gode, El Kere and Warder, where the smallpox offices were situated—and the WHO programme officers were forced to retreat. Thus, eradication activity in the area had been halted for a while. At the time, smallpox still raged on the Somali side of the border. WHO was concerned about the possibility that the smallpox in the Ogaden desert of Somalia might again be introduced to the Ethiopian side.

WHO took special countermeasures, namely the intensified surveillance for hidden foci and collection of any smallpox related information in the territories of Ethiopia, Somalia and Kenya surrounding the inaccessible fighting areas in the Ogaden. Additionally, it was fortunate that more than seventy local surveillance agents, once employed by the smallpox programme in Ethiopia, remained active in the Ogaden and continued their surveillance work, including specimen collection from suspected cases and vaccination of at-risk communities despite the fighting. These locally recruited personnel continued to communicate information and hand over specimens of suspected smallpox cases to smallpox staff in both Ethiopia and Somalia.

WHO examined and analysed in detail the surveillance information and the results of these specimens. As a result, WHO judged that there was no ongoing smallpox transmission in the Ogaden on the Ethiopian side. Why were there no cases imported from Somalia? Perhaps, it could be that the nomads living in the outbreak areas on the Somali side of the border did not have much interaction with the nomads living in Ethiopia at that time of year.

The Ethiopian army again took the Ogaden desert of Ethiopia in March 1978. I am not writing a story of warfare, but I would like to mention that this battle greatly endangered the success of the global smallpox eradication programme. For example, the Indo-Pakistan War (1970–71) resulted in a huge outbreak of smallpox in Bangladesh, with transmission of imported smallpox lasting the following three years. The Ethiopia–Somalia conflict also had the potential to bring about the resurgence of smallpox epidemics, but fortunately it did not. This fact cannot be attributed to anything else than the good luck of the programme. I should add, though, our good luck was helped considerably by the remarkable collaboration and dedication of the programme staff of Ethiopia, Kenya and Somalia to the goal of smallpox eradication. They came together irrespective of their differences in terms of politics, nationality and culture, and whether they were WHO staff or not. And, certainly, they put aside all fears regarding their own personal safety.

16

Is This the Last Case of Smallpox Globally?

In late October 1977, I visited Merca, a small port town in the south of Somalia with Zdeno Jezek. About 10 kilometres west of the town was a smallpox isolation post where three smallpox patients were being kept in isolation under the watchful eyes of the security guards.

Ali Maow Maalin, a twenty-three-year old male patient, was one of the patients to have the latest date of onset of rash on 26 October (see figure 16.1). According to my observation on 31 October, five days after the development of rash, the patient was in the late phase of vesicles with high fever.

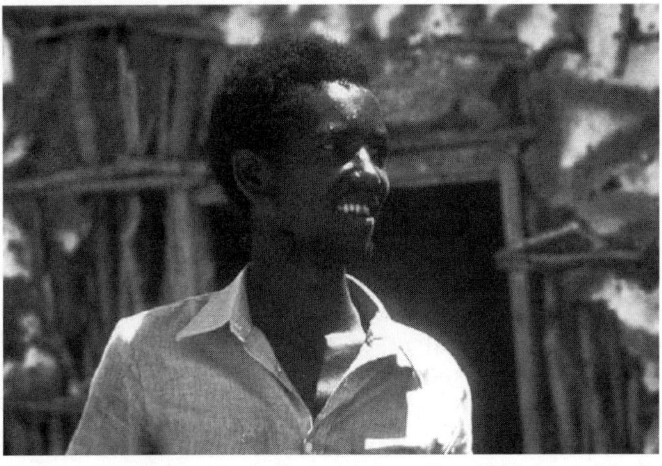

FIGURE 16.1 Last case of smallpox in Somalia: Ali Maow Maalin, 26 October 1977

Note: Ali Maow Maalin survived the infection.

Source: World Health Organization.

Jezek said, "This is the 3,229th smallpox patient in Somalia this year. The peak of the incidence was in July, and the number of patients has decreased rapidly and, therefore, this could possibly be the last patient."

To my question as to the source of the infection, Jezek replied:

> Smallpox occurred among the nomads in the desert region called Kutoware, 30 kilometres north-west of Merca. The two patients were brought here to Merca, by car, to the quarantine station at the Merca hospital.
>
> The driver could not find his way to the quarantine station at the hospital as it was dark, and he stopped on his way at the Merca hospital to ask the way to the isolation station. This patient, Ali Maow Maalin, was a cook of the hospital and in front of the hospital by chance. He got inside the car with the two patients and stayed there for only about three minutes since the quarantine station was very close. He was with them until they could find the way.
>
> As you know, we make a list of all persons who contacted patients, vaccinate them and then follow them up. However, only this patient was omitted from the list because the driver did not report this trivial matter. The hospital diagnosed his illness as malaria when he had a fever on 24 October, as the rash appeared only on 26 October, and it was not until 31 October that the patient himself suspected smallpox and a colleague at the hospital, a male nurse, reported the case to the smallpox control programme office at Merca. Notwithstanding that we took complete containment measures, we still made a mistake.

Jezek ended his narrative with a wry smile. To my query on what actions had been taken, he said, "We are carrying out a complete search for Merca residents and those who have had any contact with Merca during the time the patient was infectious". [1] The search for Merca residents was tedious work, visiting houses one by one to ask whether or not they had a fever with rash. As a result of the hard work, several patients with a fever were found, but these turned out to be not smallpox.

All the persons who had met Ali Maow Maalin, especially when he stayed at his house with a fever and rash (misdiagnosed first as suffering from malaria and then chicken pox) were examined closely.

[1] Conversation with Jezek from author's notes.

The staff and patients of the hospital in which he was admitted were also carefully examined. Eventually, a total of 161 people were examined.

This is how it was done. First, a list of contacts was prepared. Second, the smallpox programme staff visited each contact to check whether or not they had fever and rash. Third, the people on the list were not allowed to leave their homes and were in a sense quarantined. Among the 161 persons, twelve had not been vaccinated. Luckily, there were no secondary cases, perhaps because the exposure of those not vaccinated to the patient was not close enough for transmission to occur.

It was children from whom Ali Maow Maalin had got the infection. They were, as mentioned earlier, members of a nomadic family living in Kutoware, which was 30 kilometres from Merca. As it was essential to check the source of infection in that nomadic group,the enquiry revealed that these nomads were already moving north and had further divided into two or three groups.

A WHO epidemiologist, Peter Carrasco, an American, and his team immediately started tracking down the nomads. Since this area was not accessible by car, Carrasco, along with his Somali staff, organised a caravan of fourteen camels and ten donkeys to follow the family of nomads. Carrasco was usually informally dressed, wearing a T-shirt with a picture of a large butterfly, red trousers, and a hair band around his head.[2] After much effort, several days later, Carrasco and his team caught up with the group in a wild region, 70 kilometres north of Merca. A detailed investigation followed while vaccinating the family members. There were no smallpox cases, which confirmed that there had been no further spread of the virus from the two patients in the car except Ali Maow Maalin.

Jezek and I returned to Mogadishu from Merca after seeing the cases. The previously scheduled nation-wide search for smallpox cases had already begun in Somalia. We wondered if Ali Maow Maalin would be the last case. By then, the monsoon had hit Somalia. The order to strengthen the search was sent to all the programme staff

[2] In fact, another WHO staffer, who happened to see this caravan, couldn't believe his eyes when he saw the spectacle and thought that a circus had suddenly appeared in wartime Somalia.

and they struggled to reach all possible places where cases could be occurring by walking down muddy roads, riding on donkeys, and travelling in Land Rovers. Fifty Land Rovers were engaged in this difficult search, with one third of them getting stuck in the muddy roads, eventually needing to be pulled out. I returned only one time to Geneva in order to attend an important preliminary meeting of the commission for certification of smallpox eradication in Burma. The main meeting was planned for mid-November 1977.

Since Ali Maow Maalin in October 1977, no smallpox transmission has been found despite intensified searches (see figure 16.2).[3] More correctly, no endemic smallpox has been found throughout the world after Ali Maow Maalin in Somalia. However, there have been laboratory-associated smallpox cases.

At this point it is important to understand that the last case in Merca was the end point of a naturally occurring chain of transmission of smallpox that had continued for at least over 6,000 years. As for the situation surrounding the last human cases of smallpox, caused by a laboratory-associated outbreak, it is dealt with in the next chapter.

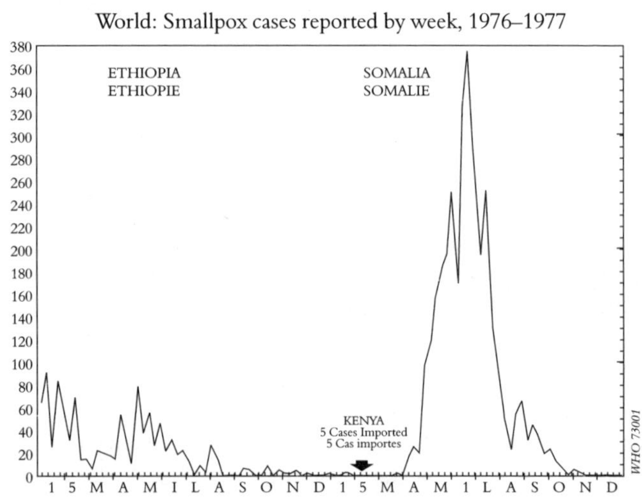

FIGURE 16.2 Horn of Africa, reported smallpox cases, by week, 1976–77

Source: World Health Organization.

[3] Up to the time of writing this book, in 2010.

17

Target Zero and Variola Virus Stocks

Infection in a Smallpox Research Institute, August 1978

Isao Arita (IA): Henry, what is the result of the diagnosis?

Henry Bedson (HB): Smallpox. Furthermore it is the virulent Asia-type.

IA: Not likely monkeypox, is it?

HB: No, it is almost without question. Our laboratory was the source of infection.

IA: ....

HB: Sorry, I remember your letter described that the functioning of a safety cabinet was suspicious, wasn't it?[1]

This is the last telephone conversation I had with the late Dr Henry Bedson, then the Director of the Virus Research Institute, Birmingham, United Kingdom, and one of the most important contributors to WHO smallpox research during the programme. Three days after the telephone conversation, he committed suicide.

In late August 1978, ten months after the last smallpox case had occurred in Somalia on 26 October 1977, I was in a telephonic conversation with a health officer of the Department of Health and Social Security, UK. The discussion went as follows:

Isao Arita (IA): A few hours ago, I heard that the suspected smallpox case worked as a medical photographer?

Health officer (HO): Yes, she belongs to the Department of Anatomy which is situated one floor above the floor of the Smallpox Research Institute of Professor Bedson, in Birmingham. She is forty years old.

[1] Author's notes.

IA: Has Mrs Parker visited the Research Institute of Dr Bedson prior to her illness?

HO: According to the investigation so far, she said that she has never been there. Furthermore, Mrs Parker only travels between her house and the Institute; she never leaves Birmingham.

IA: What kind of infection route can be assumed?

HO: Now, the UK government has set up an Emergency Committee. This committee will investigate as much as possible.

IA: I understand. That is OK. Could you tell me what is the plan on how to proceed?

HO: The illness of Mrs Parker began on 11 August 1978. The rash developed on 15 August. Smallpox was suspected on 24 August, when she was hospitalised at East Birmingham Hospital. And, when confirmed as infected with smallpox using electron microscopy, she was placed in the Isolation Hospital. Thus she is now at a quarantine station.

IA: Many days have elapsed since the onset of illness. I suppose there will be many contacts.

HO: The examination of contacts is already underway.[2]

The UK government made an all-out effort to investigate and contain the outbreak. It was ironic. Bedson had strongly contributed to the global programme since 1973, as a leading member of the Smallpox Eradication Programme of WHO. The list of his research accomplishments with smallpox virus and its analogous viruses is long. Bedson also contributed greatly through his outstanding research on monkeypox, after it was discovered in 1970 in West Africa and Zaire. Initially, there were fears that if this disease proved to be readily transmissible to humans it might mean that smallpox eradication was not feasible since there would be an animal reservoir.[3]

A group of virologists in the UK, including Professor Bedson and Keith Dumbell, provided excellent virological support to the global eradication programme and played an important role in identifying the virological features of the monkeypox virus. Professor Keith

[2] Author's notes.

[3] Monkeypox infection in humans causes a clinical picture similar to that of smallpox.

Dumbell (head of the WHO Collaborating Centre of Poxvirus Research at St Mary's Hospital Medical School London) also found a moderate type of smallpox virus (between variola major and minor, the so called intermediate type), which facilitated WHO smallpox surveillance activity. He was a good friend of Henry Bedson's. Needless to say, we were all greatly saddened by his tragic death.

As mentioned earlier, the final aim of Bedson's research was to successfully achieve the global goal of smallpox eradication. He was very pleased to hear about the last case in Somalia, with onset in October 1977. But only ten months later, Mrs Parker was infected with smallpox, with the suspected source of the infection, the smallpox viruses, kept in his laboratory. During the time, a second smallpox case occurred in the UK when the Mrs Parker's mother also contracted the disease after being infected by her daughter. Mrs Parker died on 11 September 1978. The death was broadcast across the world through international newspapers. At the time, given the possibility that some contacts of Mrs Parker might have been missed and the virus might have begun start circulating again, Bedson's chagrin can only be imagined. We assume his committing suicide was him taking responsibility for what had happened.

I now turn to laboratory-associated infection of smallpox at research institutes, a subject on which I offer some details. [4]

For a long time, people have been under an illusion that hospitals are sacred and safe places where specialists work and save lives. However, in the last dozen years or so, people have begun to realise that hospitals and research institutes too can harbour infectious diseases and can be extremely dangerous places unless appropriate countermeasures are developed to prevent such infection. Retrospectively, when we looked at data from 1961 to 1973, we found twenty-nine instances where smallpox importations caused

[4] The Birmingham laboratory-associated smallpox infection was investigated by the British government and published as a government document: *Report of the Investigation into the Cause of the 1978 Birmingham Smallpox Occurrence* (London: Her Majesty's Stationary Office, 1980). Also see, "Smallpox in Non-endemic Countries", in Fenner et al. *Smallpox and its Eradication*; and, *The Global Eradication of Smallpox: Final Report of the Global Commission for Certification of Smallpox Eradication* (Geneva: WHO, 1980).

outbreaks in Europe. Of a total of 568 cases that occurred as a result of such importations, 245 (43 per cent) were secondary cases in hospitals and among health workers. The main sources of such infections included smallpox patients who were admitted with an incorrect diagnosis, or undiagnosed smallpox cases sent for autopsy, so staff did not properly protect themselves. Although not common, hemorrhagic smallpox did occur and was difficult to diagnose correctly, even by trained physicians. In the UK, before 1978, smallpox outbreaks occurred on at least three occasions when the sources were thought to be research institutes. The first occurred in Liverpool in 1964, and the second in Midlands and Wales in 1966. The third outbreak occurred in a research institute at the London School of Hygiene and Tropical Medicine in February-March 1973, when a laboratory assistant was infected while visiting the laboratory of another department where the inoculation of smallpox virus into eggs was being done.

As for the outbreak in 1978, scientific reports indicate that there were several possibilities for the infection to have occurred at the Virus Research Institute in Birmingham. For instance, the air from the smallpox laboratory could have penetrated the whole east wing of the institute via the air ducts. While keeping the doors closed should have prevented this, it is not impossible that the doors were sometimes opened in order to use a centrifuge, incubator, refrigerator and other such equipment. The structure of the ductwork for exchanging air made it possible for airborne smallpox viruses in the smallpox laboratory to reach the darkroom where the index case (Mrs Parker) worked as a photographer. The index case also met once or twice the staff of Bedson's laboratory around late July, just when she would have been exposed to the source of infection. Thus, Mrs Parker worked all day in the room next to the smallpox laboratory, did not wear a white coat, and might not have washed her hands after finishing her work.

Three major possibilities were discussed during the investigation, but no definite conclusion was reached. The infection could have been caused by airborne spread of the viruses or else by the viruses adhering to the clothes or hands and fingers of the staff.

Fortunately, Mrs Parker retreated to her room after the onset of the disease, from 13 August to 24 August. Her visitors during this period were the primary contacts. On 24 August, Mrs Parker was moved to Saint Bartholomew's Hospital for an examination and the diagnosis was confirmed using electron microscopy. She was placed in isolation and the diagnosis was further confirmed by virus isolation on 27 August. During this period, Mrs Parker met many other patients, who were to be the secondary contacts. A total of 200 persons were identified as primary or secondary contacts. Those contacts that developed fever were sent to a quarantine ward, while other contacts were confined to their homes, until the end of the incubation period.

Mrs Parker's mother nursed her daughter from the very beginning of her illness and was therefore one of the primary contacts. Subsequently, she developed the disease in early September, within the normal incubation period for smallpox. Several of the contacts made trips to West Germany, Italy or the United States before the investigation, but all of them were contacted by the health authorities in their countries of destination and were placed under close surveillance. Vaccination was carried out on a small scale, and was mainly limited to contacts and applicants.

The vaccination history of Mrs Parker and her mother was never entirely clear. Mrs Parker was said to have been vaccinated in 1966. Probably, her mother was vaccinated in her childhood, and was revaccinated only when her daughter was diagnosed with smallpox on 24 August. However, being a close contact by then, she developed the disease before the vaccine could protect her fully.

On 16 October 1978, the British government reported the end of the outbreak at Birmingham, confirming zero secondary cases during the two-week period after the date of the complete recovery of the second case, Mrs Parker's mother.[5]

[5] The British government's official report on the matter (see footnote 4) was valuable documentation for subsequent post-eradication activities.

Assuring the Security of Variola Virus Stocks in Laboratories Globally

We again return to 1975. In late 1975, the WHO Smallpox Eradication Unit was in a new phase. In the words of D. A. Henderson: "Smallpox in the Asian Subcontinent may be finished with the last case in Bangladesh on 16 October. If this is so, there are no cases anywhere in the world, with the exception of a limited number in Ethiopia." We reviewed the possible next step.

Henderson said,

> It's time now to plan the operation of dealing with potential sources of infection at research institutes storing variola virus. It is likely that smallpox will be finished in Ethiopia within the next one or two years. Then, with the human population free from smallpox viruses, it means that only the viruses kept in research institutes will be left as a potential source of infection.
>
> The laboratory associated smallpox at the London Tropical Research Institute is a good lesson. In that case, two secondary patients died.

My response to Henderson was,

> At first, we must investigate which institutes still hold smallpox viruses. This must be a worldwide investigation, and at least eighteen months will be necessary to obtain reliable information. It is better to use a variety of methods. At first, we can request all the countries in the world to submit a report about the presence of smallpox virus. Next, we examine the medical literature for the last twenty years and make a list of all the institutes that reported studies on smallpox viruses. According to this list, we can make an inquiry to each institute as to whether or not it still holds smallpox viruses. [6]

Henderson and I agreed to adopt this plan as soon as possible, as the timing was good.

Consequently, WHO asked 181 countries to report on the presence or absence of the institutes that maintained specimens with smallpox viruses. In addition, WHO submitted a letter of inquiry to the directors of more than 200 research institutes which

[6] Author's notes.

had carried out studies on smallpox viruses and additionally about 600 virus research institutes.

The results of this investigation revealed seventy-six research institutes with smallpox viruses at the time, worldwide.

We informed these institutes that the risk associated with keeping smallpox viruses increased as the Smallpox Eradication Programme drew closer to achieving its goal of zero cases and, therefore, it was better to destroy the smallpox viruses or transfer them to a WHO collaborating institute, with the exception of special institutes that needed the viruses.

The outline of a letter from WHO sent in 1976 is reproduced here.

> Dear Sir:
>
> The Smallpox Eradication Program is gradually achieving its objective, and smallpox outbreaks are now restricted to Ethiopia. Probably, within the coming one year, the smallpox in Ethiopia will be eradicated and the day is not so far away when the number of smallpox cases will reach to zero.
>
> If smallpox disappears from the human population, it is unlikely that cases will occur again. The reasons are as follows: 1) thus far no evidence exists that smallpox viruses exist among animals, 2) the virus excretion from smallpox patients ceases within 25 days after onset of the rash, followed by no further virus excretion, and 3) smallpox viruses in the environment are inactivated within three weeks in tropical areas.
>
> On the other hand, after the disappearance of smallpox from the human population, there is some possibility that if the smallpox viruses in your institute should infect a human by mistake, the infection may lead to an outbreak of smallpox among the human population.
>
> Under the above-mentioned situation, we propose the following:
>
> If you have discontinued studies on smallpox in your institute, we would ask you to destroy the smallpox viruses as soon as possible by autoclaving them. If you wish to store your existing smallpox virus stocks, WHO will arrange for its storage at a WHO collaborating institute which has a secure storage facility.
>
> If you will continue studies with smallpox virus, we, as WHO staff, would like to know the purpose and content of the study. That is because we will need to consider whether such a study is necessary for

the promotion of the Eradication Program and eventually for human security.

We look forward to your sincere cooperation.

Best Regards[7]

Surprisingly, most of the institutes contacted and cooperated willingly and promptly. By the middle of 1977, the smallpox viruses had been removed from fifty-eight research institutes and remained stored in only eighteen.

By mid-1978, smallpox viruses had been removed from an additional six institutes, and remained in only twelve institutes. The institute where Bedson conducted his research in Birmingham was one of them and plans were made to transfer the smallpox viruses from there at the end of 1978, after conducting some more research studies. Unfortunately, shortly before the transfer of viruses could take place, Mrs Parker was infected.

Public Opinion and the Presence of the Smallpox Virus in Research Institutes

The newspapers in the UK and other European countries reported daily on the smallpox outbreak affair in Birmingham as a leading article on their front pages. This in turn aroused public discussion and safety concerns with regard to institutes storing the smallpox viruses. Consequently, most of these institutes either destroyed the viruses or transferred them to WHO-collaborating institutes with secure facilities. Only the eight institutes mentioned in table 17.1 were left with viruses in their research and storage facilities. For instance, the National Institute of Health in Japan, which used to be active as a WHO-collaborating institute, transferred its smallpox viruses to the Centers for Disease Control and Prevention, Atlanta, United States, in the autumn of 1978.

[7] World Health Organization; also see, Arita, *Smallpox Eradication*.

TABLE 17.1 Institutes storing smallpox viruses in early 1979

Country	*Institute*
USA	• Centers for Disease Control (CDC)*, Atlanta • Army Institutes for Infectious Diseases, Frederick, Maryland
UK	Saint Mary's Hospital Medical School*, London
USSR	Research Institute for Viral Preparations*, Moscow
The Netherlands	National Institute of Public Health*, Utrecht
West Germany	Institute of Tropical Medicine, Hamburg
China	Institutes for Medicine and Biological Drugs, Beijing
South Africa	National Institutes of Health, Sandringham

Note: * WHO-collaborating institutes.

In 1979, WHO called the persons in charge of the eight institutes that continued to store smallpox viruses and also the chiefs of the regulatory agencies in those countries to discuss the future plans for the viruses. Among the four institutes that were not WHO-collaborating institutes, the Army Institutes for Infectious Diseases, Frederick, Maryland, promised to transfer the virus, but the other three institutes stated that their policy was to store the virus under strict safety measures or not to destroy the virus immediately, at least at the time. However, in July of that year the Institute of Tropical Medicine in West Germany destroyed its smallpox virus samples. Further, the declaration of smallpox eradication during the World Health Assembly, 1980, lead to the reduction of the number of the laboratories retaining the variola virus (see table 17.2).

TABLE 17.2 Number of laboratories with variola virus stocks, 1979–83

	Africa	*Americas*	*Asia*	*Europe*	*Total*
1979	1	2	1	3	7
1980	1	1	1	3	6
1981	1	1	–	2	4
1982	1	1	–	1	3
1983	–	1	–	1	2

Eventually, the last two remaining laboratories holding smallpox viruses were CDC, Atlanta and Research Institute of Viral Preparations, Moscow. In fact, both continue to be WHO smallpox collaborating centres.

I describe here crucial events that took place vis-à-vis the Research Institute of Viral Preparations. At some point in the 1980s, the institute was relocated to Koltsove, Novosibirsk in Siberia. Koltsove is a town where one of the research centres for Soviet Biological Warfare Installations was located. It was generally referred to as Vector (Russian State Research Centre of Virology and Biotechnology). The installation was geared towards research, production, testing, storage, etc., in relation to biological weapons with various pathogens. The smallpox virus was of high priority among the pathogens. However, around 1991, with the collapse of the Soviet Union and setting up of a new Russian Federation, President Boris Yeltsin discontinued research of bio weapons. This is where the story gets interesting. In the same year, a high-ranking officer of the system, Kanatjan Alibekov, defected to the US where he was given a new identity and name, Ken Alibek. Ken Alibek gave a detailed description of the bio weapon research programme of the erstwhile USSR and how the smallpox virus was being used for the development of such a weapon. [8]

Thus, the extraordinary situation as regards variola virus stocks in a nation was disclosed to the notice of the West. We were uncertain how the staff of a WHO-collaborating laboratory came to be involved in such work. However, it became clear that safe management of variola virus stocks would be difficult in a post-smallpox eradication world. Subsequently, when the work associated with bio weapons declined in the Soviet Union, the variola virus was probably passed on to other countries, either through Soviet defectors or through other routes. To this day, the full extent of this spread and the locations of the virus remain unknown.

[8] D. A. Henderson, *Smallpox: The Death of a Disease* (New York: Prometheus Books, 2009).

Ken Alibek went on to publish a book on the subject of bio weapons.[9] I am uncertain of the book's accuracy; however, the implication was tragic. It meant that something tragic could happen in the future despite the success of smallpox eradication, unless we prepare well to cope with the situation in advance.

Finally, on the matter of assured security of the virus stocks, we found this to be a political issue, similar to the issue of nuclear proliferation. Appropriate and effective preventive measures require extensive research from the viewpoint of risk management. In a sense, security of the virus is related to the survival of the human species, in its evolutional process, as discussed later in the book.

[9] Ken Alibek, *Biohazard: The Chiilling True Story of the Largest Covert Biological Weapons Program in the Word; Told from Inside by the Man Who Ran It* (UK: Arrow Books, 2000).

18

Human Monkeypox: Does it Frustrate Smallpox Eradication Efforts?

In the spring of 1958, there was a commotion in the State Serum Institute, Copenhagen.[1] An outbreak of a disease similar to smallpox had occurred among Asian monkeys imported from Malaysia. Some of the monkeys had died. Until then, there had been no reports of smallpox occurring among wild monkeys. However, in 1946, an orangutan at a zoo in Jakarta developed smallpox. It is highly possible that it was infected from a smallpox patient among visitors because a large outbreak of smallpox was occurring in Jakarta at that time.[2]

Did the outbreak among the monkeys in Copenhagen represent the first known outbreak in the world of smallpox among monkeys? If it was smallpox, then Malaysia must be the source of infection since smallpox was not present in Copenhagen at the time.

On further investigation, Von Magnus and other researchers at the institute made an interesting discovery:

> The causative virus belongs to smallpox virus group, but is different from smallpox virus. Smallpox virus does not cause any change when inoculated in rabbit skin, but this virus causes necrosis in the rabbit skin. Because this virus causes smallpox-like symptoms in monkey, we will name it 'Monkeypox virus'.[3]

[1] P. Von Magnus, E. K. Anderson, K. B. Peterson and A. Birch-Anderson, "A Pox-like Disease in Cynomolgus Monkeys", *Acta Pathologica Microbiologica Scandinavica* 46, 1959, 156–76.

[2] Since monkeys resemble humans genetically, they are susceptible to smallpox. However, in monkeys, the development of the disease is different from humans.

[3] Von Magnus et al., "A Pox-like Disease".

The name "monkeypox" was eventually approved by the global virology associations. Thereafter, the monkeypox virus became a member of the pox virus group (see figure 18.1).

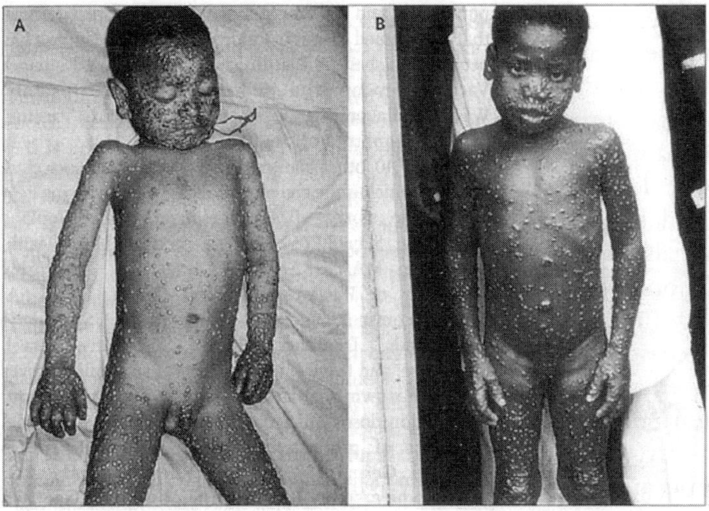

FIGURE 18.1 Similar exanthem in patients infected with (A) smallpox virus and (B) monkeypox virus on Day 7 of exanthema

Source: World Health Organization.

At the start of the smallpox eradication programme, Henderson and I were aware of the presence of monkeypox and had often discussed its implications. We both were in full agreement that the eradication programme was started based on the understanding that the smallpox virus does not exist in animals or the natural environment, and thus could be eradicated. Accordingly, we examined completely the issue of monkeypox and whether it could represent a reservoir to infect humans some time in the future.

There already was the example of the yellow fever eradication programme. We were aware that the yellow fever eradication programme was started based on a similar understanding that the causative virus occurred only in human beings. However, in the late 1920s and 1930s, when the programme was making good progress, it was found that the same virus causes the disease in monkeys living in the tropical jungles of Central and South America. Yellow fever could be transmitted from monkeys to human beings visiting the jungle through a mosquito vector. Following this discovery, eradication of the virus that causes yellow fever became impossible and the dream of yellow fever eradication had to be discarded. We knew then that we needed to investigate whether host animals for smallpox viruses existed so that we did not follow the same dead end path as the yellow fever programme.

We decided to examine thoroughly past literature on the subject in order to learn more about whether or not smallpox occurred in animals, and if so what was the present situation of the epidemiology of monkeypox.

During that summer, my family and I visited Sestri Levante, on the coast of Italy, for a three-week holiday. In the trunk of my car I packed a number of books and articles on the subject of potential animal transmission of smallpox. Although the vacation at the seaside was very pleasant, the medical literature transported me to another world and stimulated my imagination. In the literature, I found reported episodes of smallpox-like vesicular disease outbreaks in monkeys. For instance,

> In 1922, a Brazilian traveler saw that monkeys dropped from trees one by one to die. Looking at them, the whole bodies of them were covered with a rash. Around that time, an outbreak of smallpox spread like a wild fire in the town near the jungle where the monkeys were dying. [4]
>
> In 1936, Bengal, India, an outbreak of vesicular disease was observed among monkeys living in mango groves near a town and visiting the town frequently looking for food and water. The lesions were particularly in the face, palm and sole. Many died. There was no sign of smallpox in the town population despite poor coverage of smallpox vaccination. [5]

[4] I. Arita and D. A. Henderson, "Smallpox and Monkeypox in Non-Human Primates, *Bulletin of the World Health Organization* 39, 1968, 277–83. (Immediate sources of the episodes are from very old literatures, difficult to trace, hence see our references first).

[5] Arita and Henderson, "Smallpox and Monkeypox in Non-human Primates".

However, by the mid-twentieth century, reports of this kind had disappeared suddenly. Central and South America and South Asia are areas with dense populations of monkeys. With increased cultural and social activities in these regions, and therefore with the increased interaction between humans and monkeys, visitors would have encountered a continuously occurring smallpox-like disease among monkeys, in the event it occurred. Interestingly, smallpox was never reported from these regions, either among human beings or the monkeys, once human smallpox transmission had ceased. I therefore thought it possible that the occurrences in Brazil may well be another disease, for instace, a disease caused by herpes viruses.[6] However, it was possible that the disease might also be monkeypox.

I concluded that epidemiological evidence showing the occurrence of human smallpox outbreaks among wild monkeys did not exist. This fact must be true. What then was the situation of monkeypox?

Since the occurrence of monkeypox in Copenhagen in 1958, similar outbreaks among monkeys occurred in four other institutes, in Europe and North America. Interestingly, an outbreak occurring in 1964 in the zoo of Rotterdam infecting many species including gorillas, orang-utans, African green monkeys, and monkeys of Asian and African origin. However, fortunately, there were no cases reported in which humans were infected with monkeypox. Unless, of course, monkeypox outbreaks had occurred, but had gone unreported.

I must point out here that the persons working in research institutes, where there is proximity to monkeys, are well vaccinated against smallpox, and the vaccination offers prevention against both monkeypox and smallpox.

Based on this analysis, in 1968 and 1979, WHO conducted a global inquiry among institutes using monkeys as experimental animals over the occurrence of monkeypox. The inquiry resulted in an additional six outbreaks of monkeypox being discovered in institutes of Europe and North America. In the last case, a chimpanzee

[6] Some herpes viruses cause such symptoms in monkeys.

imported from Sierra Leone to Paris in 1968 was infected with monkeypox. However, all the reports were of outbreaks occurring among the monkeys in institutes, and there remained no reports of any outbreaks among wild monkeys.[7]

We continued to ask ourselves whether these findings meant that monkeypox has no relation with the smallpox eradication programme? Was the programme goal feasible?

In the autumn of 1970, while I was at the smallpox eradication unit at WHO in Geneva, I received a disturbing phone call. It was an emergency call from Dr Marennikova of the WHO collaborating institute in Moscow:

> We have just now finished the testing of a specimen from Zaire, from a 9-month old boy named Ronbe. The isolated virus is extremely similar to monkeypox virus. We will continue the investigation. But this is an important matter and thus, I have gotten in touch with you by phone immediately.[8]

According to the records available in Geneva, this patient presented smallpox-like symptoms. An operations officer of the Zaire smallpox eradication programme had taken a specimen for laboratory testing. The patient was not vaccinated, and the onset of rash occurred somewhere in the watershed region of the Zaire River (previously known as the Congo River), in Equateur province, north-west of Zaire. This is a tropical, hot and humid jungle area. It rains here for ten out of twelve months in a year. The location is very remote, taking over ten days from the capital Kinshasa, and involves travelling by airplane, jeep and canoe. Regarding smallpox in this region, the last case in the area had occurred six months previously, and no other smallpox cases were discovered until the boy was found. At the time, Ronbe was the only case of monkeypox in humans, but did his illness indicate there was a possible monkeypox outbreak in Equateur province?

[7] Arita and Henderson, "Smallpox and Monkeypox in Non-human Primates"; I. Arita, R. Gispen, S. S. Kalter, Lim Teong Wah and S. S. Marennikova, "Outbreaks of Monkeypox and Serological Surveys in Non-human Primates", *Bulletin of the World Health Organization* 46, no. 5, 1972, 625–31.

[8] Author's notes (Zaire is now termed Democratic Republic of Congo).

This concern was further strengthened by a series of events that took place in the early 1970s, which started with the WHO Reference Laboratory at CDC, Atlanta. Lets take a look at what happened.

In Liberia, the last smallpox case had occurred in 1968, in the western part of the country bordering Sierra Leone. In 1970, a telegram from CDC, Atlanta, arrived in Geneva reporting again a smallpox outbreak in mid-September in Liberia. The report indicated that the cases had occurred in an area called Chesi, located at the eastern or opposite side of Liberia from where the last case of smallpox had occurred in 1968. The area is a hot and humid tropical forest, and two cases here were diagnosed as smallpox. The cases occurred within three to four days of each other. The telegram also stated that despite the desperate efforts of the smallpox group, the source of the infection had not yet been found. Notably, Henderson, having been aware of Dr Marennikova's report on human monkeypox, advised the CDC lab staff to restudy the specimens and surveillance data.

The surrounding countries of Liberia include Sierra Leone in the west, Guinea to the north, and Cote d'Ivoire in the east. Smallpox was reported to have disappeared from all these countries. Thus, the latest smallpox outbreak raised many questions. Had there been outbreaks that were overlooked? Specimens were taken from the patients and were immediately sent to CDC, Atlanta. The initial report confirmed that smallpox-like viruses were detected. Further studies revealed surprising results with the second report confirming the virus to be monkeypox virus, the same finding as Dr Marennikova.[9]

Where smallpox viruses form white, patch-like pocks on the chorioallantoic membrane of the chick embryo, the pocks formed by monkeypox viruses become red due to bleeding. Based on this difference, the laboratory could distinguish between the two viruses. Following the finding of these monkeypox cases in humans in Liberia, human monkeypox patients were found in neighbouring countries too, with one case each found in Sierra Leone, Cote

[9] Z. Jezek and F. Fenner, "Human Monkeypox", *Monographs in Virology* 17, 1988, 1–140.

d'Ivoire and Nigeria. All these countries are located near the equator and have tropical jungle areas.

We summarised the findings so far: (a) Monkeypox viruses previously caused sporadic outbreaks among the monkeys in institutes in Europe and the USA; (b) the virus existed in the tropical forests of West and Central Africa, using as host the animals living there and only occasionally infecting human beings, as found indeed in Zaire, Liberia, Sierra Leone and elsewhere; (c) the symptoms are similar to those of smallpox, and at the time it remained unknown as to what animal carried the virus; (d) monkeys were considered to be the host or the secondary host, but rats or other animals might have also be involved, either in carrying the virus or else as the primary host.

The first problem to resolve was whether or not human monkeypox could be transmitted from human to human. A communication about human monkeypox was sent in 1971 from WHO to the countries of West Africa and Central Africa, to share available information. They were advised as follows:

> As of 1971, 9 cases of human monkeypox were found by the Smallpox Eradication Program. All the cases occurred in regions where smallpox had disappeared. The cases were sporadic and no instances of human to human transmission has been discovered. However, the symptoms are extremely similar to those of smallpox, and the causative virus is monkeypox virus belonging to the group of smallpox viruses. Please be as careful as possible regarding the occurrence of smallpox-like diseases from now on, and if cases are found or suspected please inform immediately to WHO. By the way, in the case of occurrence, please focus the epidemiological study on identifying whether or not human to human transmission is occurring. [10]

From here on, the problem of human monkeypox attracted the interest of virologists from around the world. The Smallpox Eradication Unit at WHO arranged for collection and dissemination

[10] Author's notes and WHO.

of information on epidemiological investigations and laboratory research activities on this issue.[11]

Virologists from institutes in USA, UK, Japan, France, USSR, Holland and India were involved in the research. In Liberia, Nigeria and Zaire, African mammalians, including monkeys, were captured and serum tests and virus isolation procedures conducted on them. The search for human smallpox-like diseases was also continued, after smallpox transmission in humans had stopped, in cooperation with WHO and the Government of Zaire.[12]

The following matters were clarified based on the research studies conducted at the time.

1) Forty persons suffered from monkeypox after the first patient was identified in 1970 until May 1979 (see map 18.1).
2) Among them, nine patients were from West Africa and thirty-one patients were from Zaire. In Zaire, sixteen patients were from Equateur province, and this being the largest number.
3) Two cases were likely to be the result of transmission between human beings. In the first case, in Nigeria, a mother with monkeypox was nursing a child who also developed monkeypox after ten days. In the second case, a family in Zaire, the onset of the second case, in a child, also occurred about ten days after the onset of the disease in another child. The incubation period of monkeypox (the period between the entry of virus into a host and the expression of symptoms by the host) is considered to be around ten days to two weeks and, therefore, it is highly possible that these cases were human-to-human transmission.
4) Thirty-eight patients remain after subtracting these two secondary cases from the forty cases. Among the family members who had close contact with these thirty-eight cases, and had no history of vaccination, the number of persons who could potentially have suffered from monkeypox totalled fifty-

[11] Z. Jezek, I. Arita, M. Mutombo, C. Dunn, J. H. Nakano and M. Szczeniowski, "Four Generations of Probable Person-to-Person Transmission of Human Monkeypox", *American Journal of Epidemiology*, 123, 1985, 1004–12.

[12] M. Richardson and K. Dumbell, "Comparisons of Monkeypox Viruses from Animal to Human Infections in Zaire", *Tropical and Geographical Medicine* 46, 1994, 327–29.

six. If only two patients out of the fifty-six had developed the disease, the rate of transmission from human to human was extremely low, that is two out of fifty-six, or only about 3.5 per cent. This attack rate, or rate of transmission, was only about one tenth of that for smallpox, using the figure of 35 per cent for the rate of smallpox transmission found in West Africa.

5) As mentioned above, it was thought that human monkeypox could hardly cause big outbreaks, like smallpox.
6) However, among the forty cases, six patients had died due to monkeypox, meaning that the case fatality rate was 15 per cent, about the same as that of smallpox in West Africa.
7) Many children who were not vaccinated were susceptible to the disease.

Given these findings, after detailed research and analysis, the problem of monkeypox was found to be not so much of a concern as previously thought, and did not present a risk to the theoretical basis of the Smallpox Eradication Programme. However, we could arrive at this conclusion only after the detailed research investigations and studies over a period of eight years.

Importantly, monkeypox viruses are endemic in animals living in the dense jungles of West Africa and Zaire (see map 18.1), and therefore infected human beings showing smallpox-like symptoms will continue to appear.[13] The residents in these regions have a custom of eating the meat of monkeys and rats as a source of protein, and such a custom might be the infection route of monkeypox viruses in humans. If this is the case, there is a possibility that human monkeypox might disappear provided the residents abandon such customs.

Interestingly, although vast hot and humid tropical jungles exist in a wide expanse of the equatorial areas of South America and Asia, where ecological conditions for the survival of animal viruses is considered to be not very different from those of West Africa and Central Africa, there has been no report of the occurrence of human

[13] Jezek et al., "Four Generations"; D. L. Heymann, M. V. Szczeniowski and K. Esteves, "Re-emergence of Monkeypox in Africa: A Review of the Past Six Years", *British Medical Bulletin* 54, 1998, 693–702.

MAP 18.1 Distribution of tropical rainforest and forty-four human monkeypox cases detected from 1970 to October 1979

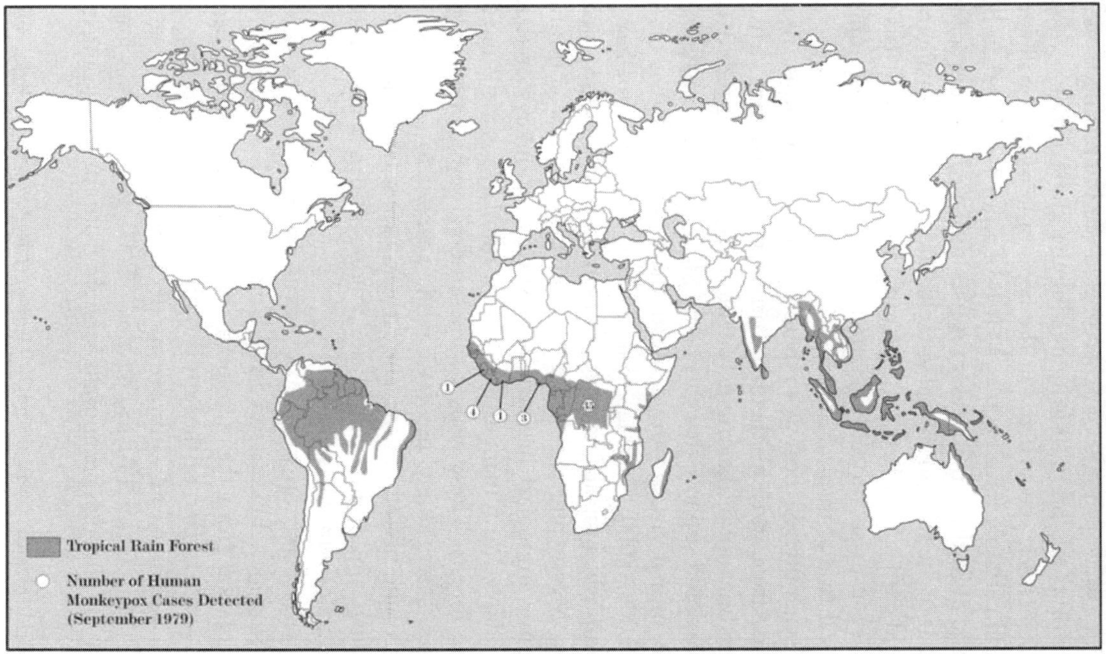

Source: World Health Organization.

monkeypox in countries such as Brazil, Indonesia, Thailand, Myanmar, and Malaysia (see map 18.1).

The story of monkeypox becomes more interesting as we think more of its evolution. It is interesting that the Australian virologist, Frank Fenner, speculated that the beginning of the smallpox virus should certainly have been as a virus of animals other than human beings, even though at present it uses the human being as its only host. If so, he said, an animal virus like the "original" smallpox virus should exist somewhere in the natural world. If such a virus exists, he said, it exists probably in the hot and humid dense jungles of tropical Asia or tropical Africa.

Fenner uttered these words before the finding of human monkeypox in Africa, and if his theory is correct, the monkeypox virus might be the burnout of the original smallpox virus he referred to.

We could suppose that there existed an "original" smallpox virus as an animal virus in the dense tropical jungles of Asia or Africa, say 5,000–6,000 years ago. Part of the "original" smallpox virus accomplished the adaptation to human hosts to become a smallpox virus. Meanwhile the "original" smallpox viruses continued to transmit among its original hosts such as monkeys or rats, and also adapted to remain as the present monkeypox virus in African native forests. These viruses sometimes cause infection in human beings. Interestingly, however, while adapted to monkeys or rats over a long period of time, the virus does not have the capacity to establish continuous transmission among human beings although it can infect them sporadically.

The research on monkeypox virus not only directly benefited the Smallpox Eradication Programme, but also provided useful information from the standpoint of the developmental theory of pathogens. In fact, further study on the subject is expected.

In recent years, human monkeypox outbreaks have been reported in Central Africa.[14] Also, in 2003, the virus was imported to the US through pet animals brought from Africa, causing human

[14] World Health Organization, "Human Monkeypox in Kasai Oriental, Democratic Republic of the Congo (former Zaire): Preliminary Report of October 1997 Investigation", *The Weekly Epidemiological Record* 72, 1997, 369–72.

monkeypox outbreaks. None of these later cases revealed new findings, which necessitated changes to the recommendations of the WHO Commission for the Certification of Smallpox Eradication, including that monkeypox surveillance should be continued.[15]

During the surveillance activities for monkeypox, there were two episodic events that could, in retrospect, be interesting for readers. The first one was the abduction of a child by a chimpanzee in East Zaire; the child was soon recovered, but after sustaining a superficial wound on the leg. She developed a typical monkeypox rash thirteen days after the incident and the monkeypox virus was isolated. Although the chimpanzee was confirmed as not infected with the monkeypox virus, it was considered to be an example of monkey-to-person virus transmission.[16] The second incidence was a history of the isolation of a smallpox-like virus during the passage of monkeypox or simple monkey kidney cell cultures at the laboratory. The incidence caused a great deal of concern and studies were conducted to elucidate the true nature of the virus isolate as such. It was tentatively termed white poxvirus (details are discussed in box 18.1). I personally believe it could have been a laboratory contaminant. This incident shows that even a good laboratory can cause contamination and, further, the fact that the workers in the smallpox eradication were serious to determine any doubtful phenomena.

Box 18.1 Whitepox virus mystery

One day, Svetlana Marennikova came to meet me at the WHO office in Geneva. She looked a bit exhausted and worried, perhaps due to her heavy workload. She was the director of the WHO Collaborating Center on Smallpox and Poxviruses, Moscow, and an eminent poxvirus virologist. She was also the first expert to identify human monkeypox cases.

[15] The WHO Global Commission for the Certification of Smallpox Eradication, Geneva, did so in 1980.

[16] M. G. Mutombo, I. Arita and Z. Jezek, "Human Monkeypox Transmitted by a Chimpanzee in a Tropical Rain-Forest Area of Zaire", *Lancet* 321, no. 8327, 1983, 735–37.

She told me that during her recent work making passages of monkeypox virus in her lab, she had made a chance discovery of white pock lesions on the chorioallantoic membranes of the chick embryo. According to her, they bore a strong resemblance to smallpox. On her second attempt to try and identify the sample as variola or monkeypox virus, she was still unable to differentiate the sample from variola virus. As I remember, she had visited me some time late in the 1970s, just when we were hoping to shortly finish the eradication programme.

Thus, we were worried. As mentioned earlier in the chapter, yellow fever eradication had failed. Did the Moscow report indicate a similar fate for smallpox? We were worried. At that time, in fact, including the isolates in Moscow, we had at least sixteen isolates of unclear origin, but resembling the phenotype of variola virus: they were termed as white poxvirus, white clone or white mutant. Thus we organised special research involving WHO smallpox reference laboratories in Moscow, Bilthoven (the Netherlands), London and Atlanta

Keith Dumbell in London and J. J. Esposito and J. H. Nakano, Atlanta, joined the team carrying out extensive genetic studies to find out the nature of white poxvirus. The results were fascinating: of the sixteen isolates under study, DNA analysis showed that the variola viruses were not mutants of the monkeypox virus or vice versa.[17] These research results contributed to our confidence that there was little risk of smallpox returning from nature after eradication. The results also highlighted the possibility that laboratory contamination can occur even in the most stringent laboratories. At the beginning of the intensified programme, many scientists said that smallpox was a simple disease, and that no research was needed. However, this episode teaches us the lesson that for every programme, no matter how simple it may appear, research is always an important component. Over the last three decades, without any vaccination programme, there has not been a single case of smallpox.

[17] K. R. Dumbell and L. C. Archard, "Comparison of White Pock (h) Mutants of Monkeypox Virus with Parental Monkeypox and with Variola-like Viruses Isolated from Animals", *Nature* 286, no. 5768, 1980, 29–32; J. J. Esposito, J. H. Nakano and J. F. Obijeski, "Can Variola-like Viruses be Derived from Monkeypox Virus? An Investigation Based on DNA Mapping", *Bulletin of the World Health Organization* 63, 1985, 695–703.

19

Has Smallpox Really Gone? How Do We Know?

To doubt is to become clever. Science does not advance without doubt. In the case of eradication, it is natural to be suspicious, especially if the question concerns the removal of smallpox. There have been several widely held observations on the matter. Most important of these is the one which asks how to ascertain that smallpox does not exist in areas inaccessible due to geographical, political or security-related reasons. Ahead, I discuss some such interesting communications the WHO received from various quarters.

Early in the 1970s, while the smallpox eradication programme was ongoing, a professor from the US wrote to the WHO:

> I was invited by some university in the Middle East to give a lecture. As I was interested in WHO smallpox eradication, I talked about this programme. After the lecture, a few students came up to me and said: 'You said there is no smallpox in the Middle East. This is not true; we have smallpox in our country.' I advise WHO to investigate this report. [1]

Following up on this communication, we discovered that the students were actually correct. This was one of the positive rumours. There were of course several false reports too. It was difficult to say when a report was positive or false, until we had investigated it fully.

I recall how in 1977 a press report in the Philippines reported smallpox outbreaks on Mindanao Island, resulting in over ten deaths. The news spread worldwide through the press in the Americas,

[1] Author's notes.

Europe and East Asia (it later turned out, on further investigation, that the report was false, as mentioned at the end of the chapter).

A few professors at the Academy of Sciences in France were suspicious of WHO's claims of smallpox eradication. An extract of their letter to WHO follows.

> Director-General,
>
> WHO indicated the requirements for verification of smallpox eradication in many Asian countries in its *Weekly Epidemiological Report* dated 13 January 1978. But the article mentioned nothing regarding smallpox in Siberia, Korea and Japan. We would like to know how it was possible to determine that there is no smallpox transmission in such areas, inaccessible due to geographical, political, or security related reasons such as the Amazon basin, Himalayas, Tibet and terrorist camps.
>
> The US and UK discontinued smallpox vaccination, having believed the WHO smallpox reports: it is worrisome.[2]

In 1978, we received the following report from Australian travellers:

> We were asked for our international certificates of smallpox vaccination. WHO said there is no smallpox in Asia? Why did they ask for our certificates? Perhaps they have cases of smallpox since when we waited for the ferry, we saw a man covered full with smallpox-like eruptions. How have reports by every nation been accurate?[3]

Even some WHO staff members commented on their doubts:

> In a slum in Calcutta, more than nineteen people are living in one room; a town with narrow roads of 1 metre. The smallpox goddess is still worshipped. How do you know smallpox patients are not hiding in such a place? You know, on the planet, if we have one smallpox case, there will be another patient, and then another. How is it possible to say there is no smallpox?[4]

All these comments or rumours were in fact helpful for the WHO smallpox eradication programme. We took every single rumour

[2] Author's notes.

[3] Ibid.

[4] Ibid.

and report seriously, investigated it and identified the area of risk wherever possible. For example, the Government of the Philippines confirmed that the 1977 Mindanao Island outbreak had been a false rumour, after a team investigated the area using a helicopter.

How did WHO handle this issue of no further smallpox outbreaks? How did it ascertain, in a given region, that smallpox had indeed been eradicated? What WHO did was systematically intensify smallpox surveillance activities as the eradication programme progressed, in the context of verification of no smallpox report. Let us now return to 1971, at a somewhat earlier stage of the programme.

In 1971, the WHO Global Commission for the Certification of Smallpox Eradication met and discussed the definition of smallpox eradication. It was decided that, "The only smallpox virus reservoir is man, hence zero cases in the population is eradication". The difficulty lay in determining what could be the "last case". For instance, in Nigeria, there occurred a smallpox case six months after WHO had thought they had seen the last smallpox outbreak! Could the following be analysed: the length of time between the month when a national programme announced its last smallpox case and the date of the real last case?

Finally, the WHO Global Commission for the Certification of Smallpox Eradication decided to establish a provisional timetable of the requirements for smallpox surveillance. It was to be maintained at a high level for a period of two years following the last case before a programme could declare freedom from smallpox.[5] Further, the WHO Global Commission expanded the conditions beyond the country level: 1) if such a condition is fulfilled in a continent or WHO region, we can certify that the continent or WHO region has become smallpox free; 2) if such situation is accomplished in all regions and continents, we can say that global smallpox eradication has been accomplished.

This was the definition, or concept, of certification of smallpox eradication. Based on this concept in principle, the certification

[5] The experience in Indonesia was noted, where eight months had elapsed between the date of onset of the assumed last case and the date of onset of the real last case.

of smallpox eradication started in a few WHO regions and finally reached the global certification of smallpox when all WHO regions had been certified. As shown in table 19.1, the first certification was conducted in the region of South America, in 1973, two years after the date of the last smallpox case in 1971 in Brazil. A similar procedure followed in other regions or countries where regional committees had been formed by the WHO. Each committee consisted of selected experts as well as health officers. Individual regions or groups of countries in need of the certification were investigated by their respective committees. The committees on their part checked the country's records and epidemiological situation in previous smallpox affected areas. The certification work covered seventy-nine countries from 1973 to 1979, as indicated in table 19.1. The certification committees were in fact the best available experts specifically requested by WHO. They faced a mammoth task, but it was with a sense of global responsibility that they went about it, for the results dramatically impacted world health security.

The last certification of zero cases worldwide was made exactly two years after the last case occurred in Somalia, on 26 October 1979. The validity of this certification work can be considered solid because there has been no smallpox reported in the world for almost three decades since the declaration of smallpox eradication in 1980 by the World Health Assembly (WHA). Notably, at the 1980 WHA, delegates of all member states signed the document indicating freedom from smallpox in their own nations. Parenthetically, I should mention that even though table 19.1 looks rather cumbersome, it illustrates the enormous work of verification of the epidemiological information done by individual nations, as well as the certification committees listed here. The table was taken as it is from the final report of the Global Commission for the Certification of Smallpox Eradication, WHO, published in 1980.

TABLE 19.1 Seventy-nine countries requiring special certification procedures, year of last smallpox and of certification

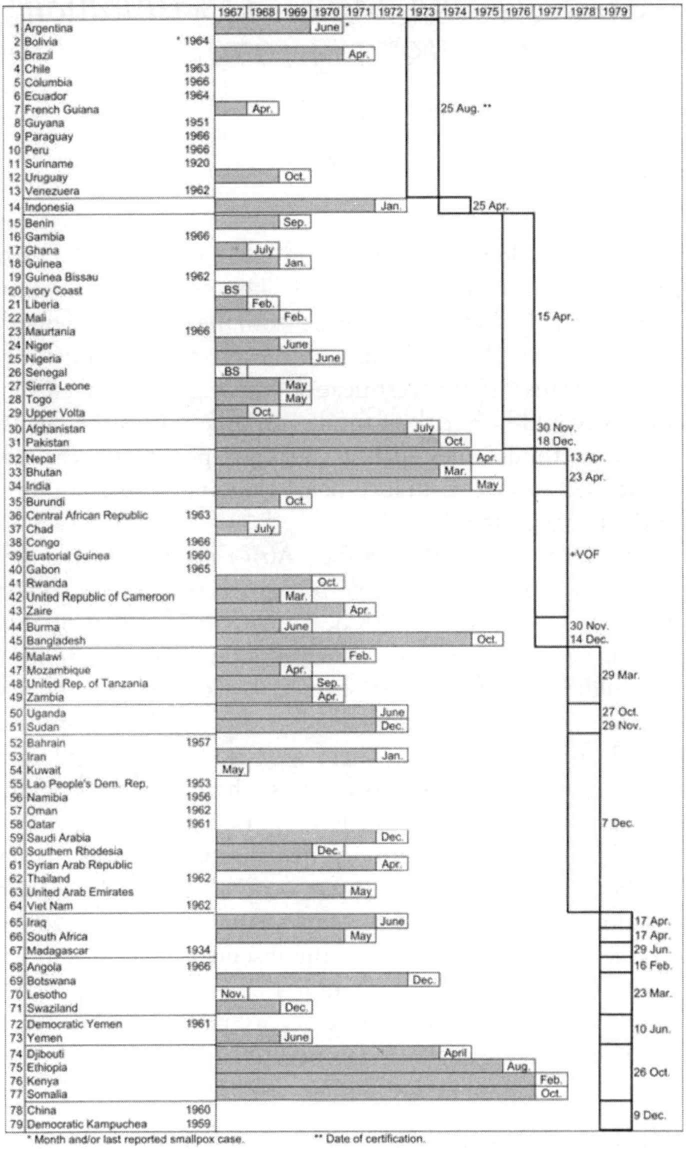

Source: World Health Organization.

20

Strategies and Tactics of Certification, 1973 to 1979

The WHO Smallpox Eradication Unit had to use several innovative approaches in the certification process. The certification committees always included a few health officers from the countries which were located in geographic proximity to the group of countries being certified because if the certification findings proved false, their countries would be at risk of future importations of the disease. In addition, methodologies such as smallpox pockmark scar surveys were utilised to give assurance of no ongoing smallpox outbreaks after the last reported case.

In western Africa—the part of Africa which became free of smallpox in 1971—an extensive pockmark survey was conducted in primary school children to detect any hidden foci of recently occurring cases (figure 20.1). Of 6.5 million people examined (half were children), 8,600 people showed pockmarks, but they were all estimated to have been infected prior to 1970, before the last reported case in the region. There were no children aged younger than six years with pockmarks. Thus, there was no evidence of smallpox transmission after the last reported case in Nigeria.

In Afghanistan, the committee investigations included a review of the activity of variolators. It was concluded that the practice of variolation had been stopped a few years before the certification team visit, presumably because of the absence of smallpox materials. In Pakistan, varicella (or chickenpox) cases were studied in large numbers by the national laboratory as part of rash with fever surveillance. The results were all negative for smallpox during the two-year certification period. In India and Bangladesh, nation-wide active searches for hidden smallpox cases were conducted at least three times in India and eight times in Bangladesh after the last reported case. Also, in both countries, the reward for reporting smallpox cases was increased. The reward for reporting a new smallpox case was Rs 1000 in India and 1000 taka in Bangladesh, substantial sums of money for the average person. Surveys showed that the reward was known to almost 80 per cent of villagers in India. In fact, an amusing joke did the rounds at the time, that the smallpox reward was better known to the villagers in India than the name of the then prime minister Indira Gandhi! Eventually, based on these activities, the WHO South-East Asia Region was certified to be smallpox free by December 1977.

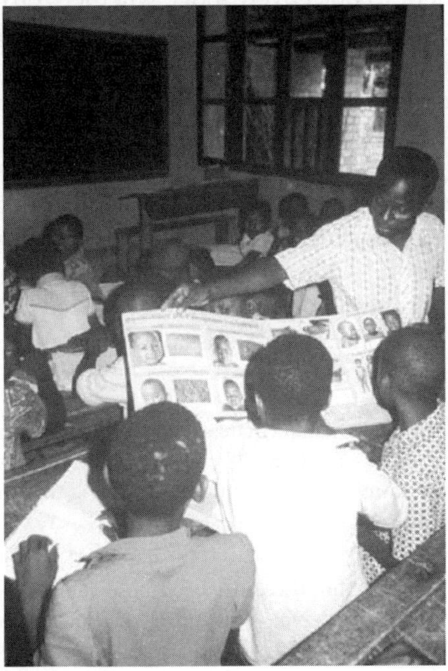

FIGURE 20.1 Active search for smallpox in school

Source: World Health Organization.

The year 1977 was a busy one for the global smallpox eradication programme. The certification process mentioned above was making rapid progress, while, simultaneously, a smallpox outbreak was being controlled in Somalia. Following the onset of the last case on

26 October 1977, the two-year certification process was initiated in the Horn of Africa. In October of the same year, WHO held at its headquarters, Geneva, the meeting of the Global Commission for the Certification of Smallpox Eradication to discuss how to eliminate the probable last endemic smallpox in the Horn of Africa and simultaneously proceed with the global certification process. The commission consisted of experts from nineteen countries, particularly those individuals who had led the Horn of Africa programmes.

At the time, I was convinced that although the commission had to be independent to objectively judge whether zero incidence had been achieved, some of the members also had to be familiar with the eradication programme to fully assess the work done. Even persons involved in the actual eradication programme could fully satisfy the criteria of independence since all members knew that eradication was a historically unprecedented event in medicine and its judgement posed a grave responsibility on all participants. Similarly, the WHO smallpox eradication staff also felt the responsibility to reach the correct conclusions.

The Global Commission meeting was chaired by Frank Fenner. The salient points of the discussions and deliberations are described in the following extracts:

> Of close to 200 WHO member states, 79 needed special measures, such as certification commission visits. The rest of the countries were required by the commission to submit statements certifying that there had been no recent smallpox cases (In fact, these statements were submitted to the WHA in 1980).
>
> Unlike influenza or polio, there has been no evidence of the presence of any poxvirus illnesses having smallpox-like clinical pictures. During an age when European explorers sailed around the world 400 years ago, the smallpox virus spread to the Americas, to the Pacific islands and elsewhere with no evidence of genetic changes. This would suggest, there has been no evidence that the smallpox virus is not stable and capable of changing its features of current pathogenicity.
>
> There has been no evidence of the existence of animal reservoirs of the smallpox virus, other than man.
>
> The risk of smallpox virus in specimens from dead and buried smallpox cases in the cold weather areas, and even variolators' specimens kept in

> Afghanistan mountainous area, needed to be checked. Of 21 specimens from Afghanistan studied, including crusts, it was revealed that the virus did not survive after 10 months time. Already five years have elapsed since the date of the last smallpox case in Afghanistan. I am reflecting now in 2009, that while the risk may appear to be negligible, we may need more time on this issue not only in relation to Afghanistan but also any cold climate area with sub-freezing temperatures. However, S. Marennikova in her studies once tried and failed to revive the virus from specimens from smallpox cases that had become unfrozen due to warming climate. [1]

After deliberating over several issues, it was unanimously agreed that the following two were most important: (a) to confirm that no smallpox occurred in human beings at the global level and (b) to prevent the escape of the smallpox virus from the research institutions where stocks still remained for studies. There was a strong proposal from virologists that smallpox research be continued, as there still remained many ambiguous points.

The Global Commission meeting finally recommended the following:

1. The certification committee should be called the Global Commission for Certification of Smallpox Eradication and that it would meet again the following year, in December 1978, to assess progress.
2. All efforts should be made to stop smallpox transmission in the Horn of Africa, as that could result in global eradication of smallpox.
3. The laboratories with smallpox virus stocks should be limited to those designated by WHO as WHO collaborating laboratories for smallpox.
4. A smallpox vaccine stockpile of 300 million doses should be retained for any possible emergency.

Following the conclusions by the Global Commission, special efforts took place for the completion of the global smallpox eradication programme. I draw your attention to the salient activities during the period, 1978–79.

[1] Arita, *Smallpox Eradication*, 193–98.

In May 1978, when the World Health Assembly (WHA) promulgated the US $1000 smallpox reward (figure 20.2) to the reporter of any new case of smallpox anywhere in the world, I was surprised by the large number of reports we received at the WHO office in Geneva from different parts of the world. The WHO smallpox staff carefully studied every report. Many were found to be varicella or other exanthemata diseases; some were false alarms. None gave any confirmed evidence of smallpox.

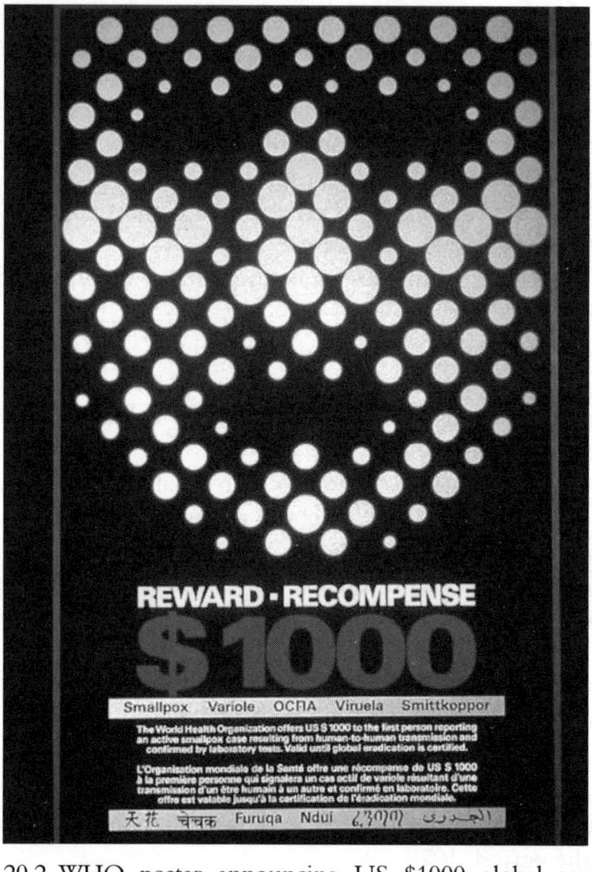
REWARD · RECOMPENSE
$1000
Smallpox Variole ОСПА Viruela Smittkoppor
The World Health Organization offers US $ 1000 to the first person reporting an active smallpox case resulting from human-to-human transmission and confirmed by laboratory tests. Valid until global eradication is certified.
L'Organization mondiale de la Santé offre une récompense de US $ 1000 à la première personne qui signalera un cas actif de variole résultant d'une transmission d'un être humain à un autre et confirmé en laboratoire. Cette offre est valable jusqu'à la certification de l'éradication mondiale.
天花 चेचक Furuqa Ndui الجدري

FIGURE 20.2 WHO poster announcing US $1000 global reward for reporting a smallpox case, 1978–79

Source: World Health Organization.

During 1978–79, of the seventy-nine countries to be certified, forty-five had been certified as free of smallpox; however, thirty-four countries still awaited certification. This group included countries that were not in contact with the UN due to national policy or some difficult political situation. For instance, Zimbabwe (then Rhodesia) was only recognised by the UN in 1980. There had therefore been no WHO assessment of the smallpox situation there. Gordon Meiklejohn[2] (of the US) and Nicole Grasset (WHO staff) visited Rhodesia in February 1978. They travelled guarded by the army due to possible guerrilla attack. The available surveillance data, as well as the visit of the WHO team to the area where the last smallpox case was found in April 1972, all indicated that there was no ongoing transmission of smallpox since the date of the occurrence of the reported last case. On return to Geneva, they reported complete absence of smallpox, adding that the real worry had been the explosion of a mine at anytime during their field trip!

At that time, a few other countries also faced similar problems with certification. But, surprisingly, and sometimes with great luck, we were able to accomplish the task. South Africa and Namibia wholeheartedly collaborated with WHO for the certification investigations. Angola helped the WHO team travel safely and without restriction. In Uganda, the then president himself made arrangements for the team and gave them a free hand to conduct their investigations. Many African nations tried to help with their limited resources available. Iran collaborated despite the pre-revolution confusion prevailing in the state.

In Asia, Cambodia was in the midst of a civil war. The then national government submitted its report declaring the state rid of smallpox while in exile; ironically, it made this declaration while another government, not recognised by the UN, was controlling the health system of the country. It was therefore not possible to certify eradication with such an external report. It was pure chance that one WHO staff met, by chance, an official from Cambodia and he assisted in preparation of the true report based on the situation

[2] A professor of internal medicine at Denver University. During his sabbatical year, he came to Geneva to help with smallpox eradication as a WHO consultant.

in Cambodia. The report provided sufficient proof that there was no smallpox there.

China showed initial reluctance in collaborating with the certification effort due to a misunderstanding that the process would mar the state's national pride at achieving long time freedom from smallpox since the 1960s. Finally, owing to the help of Gustav Nossal (from Australia), the government accepted the visit of a WHO team comprising Frank Fenner and Joel Breman. In July 1979, the WHO team travelled to several provinces in China, including the two provinces bordering India and the province with the last reported smallpox case; the team also covered several countries in Indochina. They conducted pockmark surveys in at-risk areas where the last smallpox cases were reported in 1960 and 1961. The team also examined the records of the smallpox programme, including data on variolation sometime in the early 1960s. There was no evidence of endemic smallpox in China since 1961. The only concern in Fenner's report, as I recall now, was that there had been cases caused by variolation in the northern part of China, in Shanxi province, with four cases in 1965. This, however, had occurred well before the visit of certification team, over fourteen years earlier, and was therefore not seen as a problem. I recount it here for the interested reader.

It should be mentioned that all countries welcomed the certification process and work involved. I believe that it is this close and friendly collaborative effort between the countries and respective certification committees that contributed to the success of the programme (see map 20.1). Collaboration between countries was a characteristic of the eradication programme and it contributed to the programme's success. In the next chapter, I will discuss how the certification process proceeded in the Horn of Africa. Since it was the final effort to complete the intensified programme, some additional details, as seen from my perspective at the time, are described.

Map 20.1 Year of certification, by country

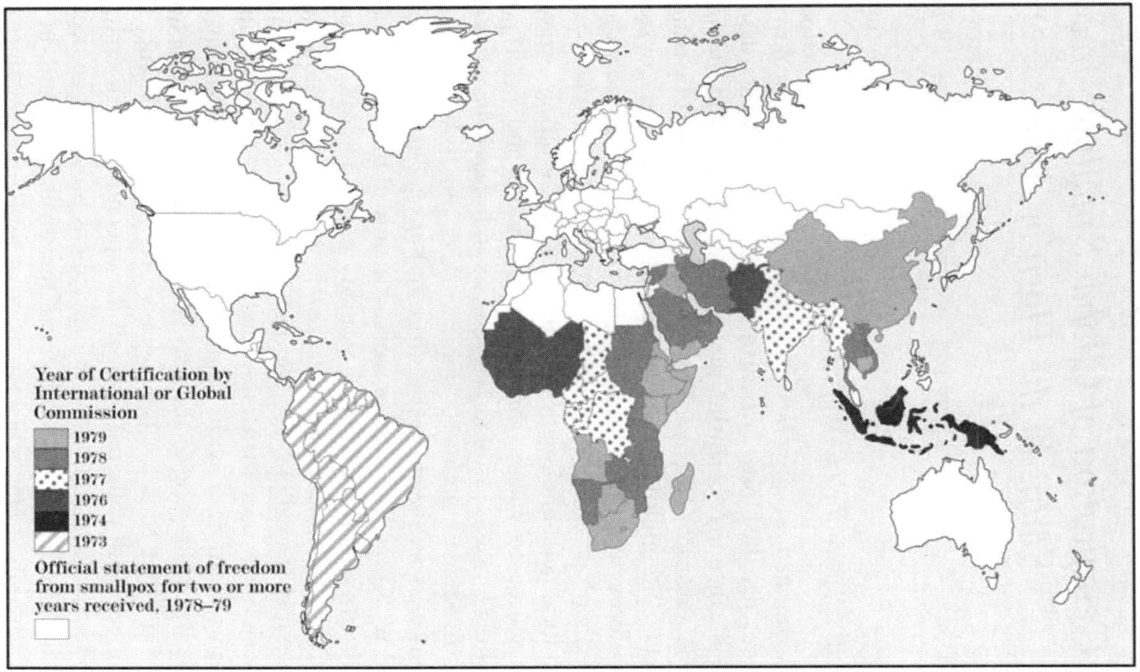

Source: World Health Organization.

21

Certification of Global Smallpox-free Status in the Horn of Africa

Special Effort in the Horn of Africa

As mentioned in previous chapters, smallpox outbreaks were discovered in the Horn of Africa in 1976, first in the Ogaden desert in Ethiopia, then in Mogadishu, the capital of Somalia, and later in the Mandera district of Kenya. The extensive joint efforts by national, bilateral and multilateral organisations succeeded in containing the outbreak and finding the last case in Somalia, probably the last naturally occurring case of smallpox on earth. In Ethiopia, around 1,000 local personnel, with four WHO medical officers, travelled from village to village, through mountainous and desert areas, searching for cases. Around 100 vehicles and a few helicopters were used. In Somalia, about 700 local workers and 10 WHO medical officers were employed in the effort. In Kenya, 200 local personnel and 2 WHO medical officers worked mainly in the northern areas where Ethiopian and Somali nomads used to travel. Djibouti, adjacent to Ethiopia and Somalia, also intensified the search for any hidden foci of smallpox (see figures 21.1 and 21.2).

In all areas, specimens were collected from cases of patients suffering from rash with fever, suspected to be smallpox, and dispatched for testing to the two WHO collaborating laboratories in Atlanta and Moscow (see figures 21.1 and 21.2). Some 2,900 specimens were collected from all the operational areas each year in 1978 and 1979 and tested. All specimens proved to be negative for smallpox. The announcement of the smallpox reward, in May 1978, certainly strengthened reporting of smallpox cases, since such a reward system was well known in the population of the regions, even among nomadic populations.

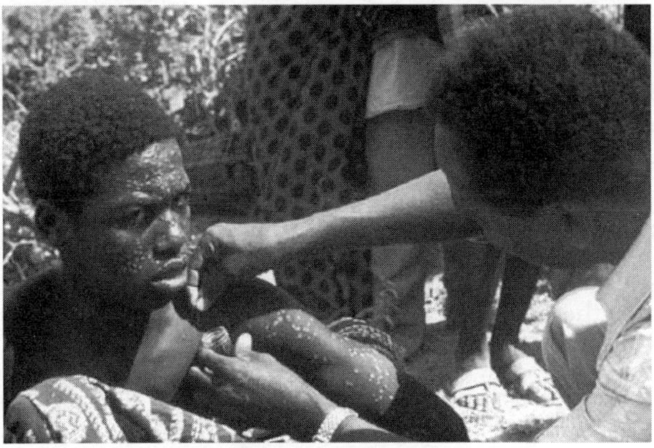

FIGURE 21.1 Specimen collection, Africa

Note: Educational slide pictures distributed by WHO to all African country programmes showing specimen collection from a smallpox patient for its laboratory confirmation in 1977–79.

Source: World Health Organization.

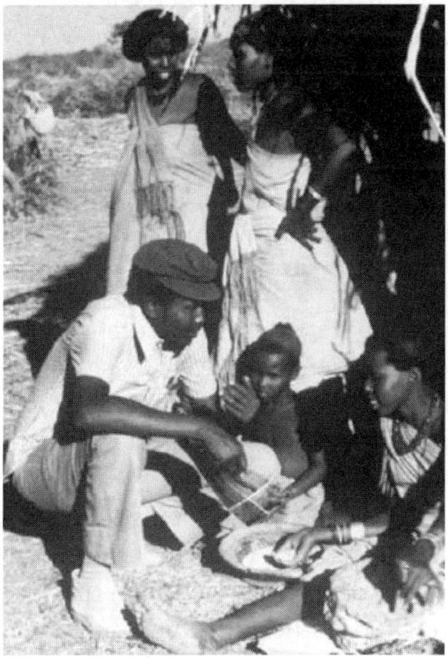

FIGURE 21.2 A surveillance agent questions nomad women in Somalia

Source: World Health Organization.

The WHO Global Commission for the Certification of Smallpox Eradication visited four countries in the Horn of Africa from 1 to 20 October 1979 Thereafter, they met at Nairobi, reviewed the results of their investigations, including both surveillance records and actual visits to areas with the last cases, and then zeroed in on areas at highest risk of continuing smallpox transmission. The Global Commission discussed its findings at this Nairobi conference and finally concluded that there was no evidence of any further smallpox cases since the last reported case two years earlier. The day was 26 October 1979, two years since the date of onset of smallpox rash of the last case discovered in Somalia.

World Health Assembly, 1980

On 8 May 1980, the World Health Assembly (WHA) accepted the following conclusions of the Global Commission: (i) that smallpox eradication has been achieved throughout the world; and (ii) that there is no evidence that smallpox will return as an endemic disease. Accordingly, the following statement of the WHA resolution 33.3 was prepared:

> [The WHA] Declares solemnly that the world and all its peoples have won freedom from smallpox, which was a most devastating disease sweeping in epidemic form through many countries since earliest times, leaving death, blindness and disfigurement in its wake, and which only a decade ago was rampant in Africa, Asia and South America.

Was it an impossible statement? In actual fact, this statement was a revised one. I was present at the WHA session and will recount what really went on. Some of these incidents are most enjoyable! First, when the prepared statement was presented, the WHA delegate from USSR was most dissatisfied with the end result and declared, "this is not adequate to mark this unprecedented event. Please make it more impressive!" The WHA statement, eventually made public, is the revised second statement urgently prepared by James Magee, an able WHO smallpox unit consultant information officer, who was handling publicity in the final stage of the programme. He was a former reporter from the UN Press Club.

Thus, the WHA declaration of the eradication of smallpox and the recommendation to discontinue smallpox vaccination means the epoch-making end of a global programme. I was asked by many reporters as well as scientists how I felt about the end of this programme. Certainly I was most pleased, but frankly speaking I felt nothing special except for instinctively feeling that we would start the post-eradication activities, which would be continued as an inseparable programme from the so far conducted smallpox eradication enterprise. There were also a few projects to complete in the programme such as the documentation of the programme development and results, archiving or preservation of programme records and artefacts, and, most importantly, the immediate planning of how to prevent any possibility of the return of the smallpox virus to human populations. This last point related to dealing with the variola virus retained in laboratories and the possibility of its deliberate release. These projects were all recommended in the final report of the Global Commission of the Certification of Smallpox Eradication, WHO 1980. The Commission also recommended WHO to maintain the core group of epidemiologists at its headquarters in Geneva. In fact, I stayed in Geneva with a few of my long-time colleagues until April 1985, when I said goodbye to WHO and left for Japan.

Before discussing post-eradication in the next two chapters, I would like to narrate some episodic stories directly related to the so far conducted eradication operations in this chapter, instead of a concluding opinion of an unprecedented event in public health history. Therefore, I discuss here some conference and episodic events that occurred after the declaration of smallpox eradication on 8 May 1980. I hope readers will understand the reason behind my writing in this way.

Dahlem Conference, Berlin, 1997

The best recollection and analysis of the smallpox eradication programme would be to mention the Dahlem Workshop Conference, which was held in Berlin almost two decades after eradication was achieved, in 1997. About forty participants (including those who had first-hand experience in smallpox eradication) met and discussed experiences and prepared a report, which would be useful for those interested in disease eradication.[1] It covered pertinent elements of disease eradication such as definition, management, microbiology, epidemiology, and socio-economic aspects with special focus on the successful smallpox eradication programme and the lessons learned from the programme. I was also one of the speakers at the workshop. Figure 21.3 formed an important part of my presentation, for global eradication as a logical consequence of the evolution of medical technology—the mainstream of globalisation—which had started in the late twentieth century and is continuing in the twenty-first century. Note that this is contrasted by the revival in the trend of individualisation on the other extreme end.

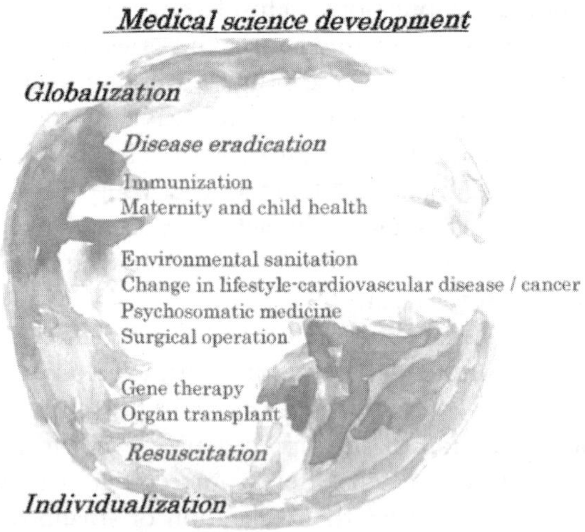

FIGURE 21.3 Medical science development

Bill Foege also attended the workshop and spoke on "Thoughts on organization for disease eradication". He stressed that eradication

[1] I. Arita, "Are There Better Global Mechanisms for Formulating, Implementing, and Evaluating Eradiation Programs?" *The Eradication of Infectious Diseases: Report of the Dahlem Workshop on the Eradication of Infectious Diseases*, Berlin, March 16–22, 1997, ed. W. R. Dowdle and D. R. Hopkins (New York: John Wiley & Sons, 1998), 176–86.

did not require any elaborate and large-scale organisation, but rather a small and effective core group that adjusts strategy and allows for coordinated implementation whenever required. Also, a point I stressed during the workshop was that eradication must be completed within ten to fifteen years. Any eradication programme needs uniform development by both the rich and the poor and such a condition cannot be sustained over a long period. As shown in map 21.1, there have been (and continue to be) a number of countries in sub-Saharan Africa and South Asia suffering from extreme poverty, where increased levels of health resources are needed even if only for several years to accomplish the globally uniform implementation of the eradication strategy. Thus the prolonged eradication time factor tends to result in the failure of global eradication. In this respect, the bilateral collaboration by the USA in the initial smallpox eradication efforts in nineteen countries of West and Central Africa was the important factor that contributed to the global success of smallpox eradication.

Foege ended his talk saying the discussion on eradication moved beyond the issue of disease: "If eradication efforts are successful, they contribute to the improvement of civilization and necessary experience base that will be required for global peace".[2] At the time, Foege's talk reminded me of some unusual occurrences during the implementation of the smallpox programme, narrated ahead.

During the Indian autumn campaign, D. A. Henderson (in the Geneva office) suddenly received a call from Dr V. T. H. Gunaratne, Regional Director of the WHO Regional Office for South-East Asia in New Delhi, who was angry with one of the smallpox staff from Geneva, stationed at the regional office. This staff wanted to fly to Nepal following a report of smallpox cases, but the Regional Director's approval was delayed. The smallpox staff became impatient and wrote a note about the delay to the WHO smallpox unit in Geneva. Unfortunately, the note was inadvertently dropped in the corridor of the regional office. Somebody picked it up, and and handed over the note to the office of the Regional Director.

[2] W. Foege, "Thought on Organization for Disease Eradication", in Dowdle and Hopkins, *The Eradication of Infectious Diseases*, 187–92.

MAP 21.1 Nations below US $600 of GNI per capita

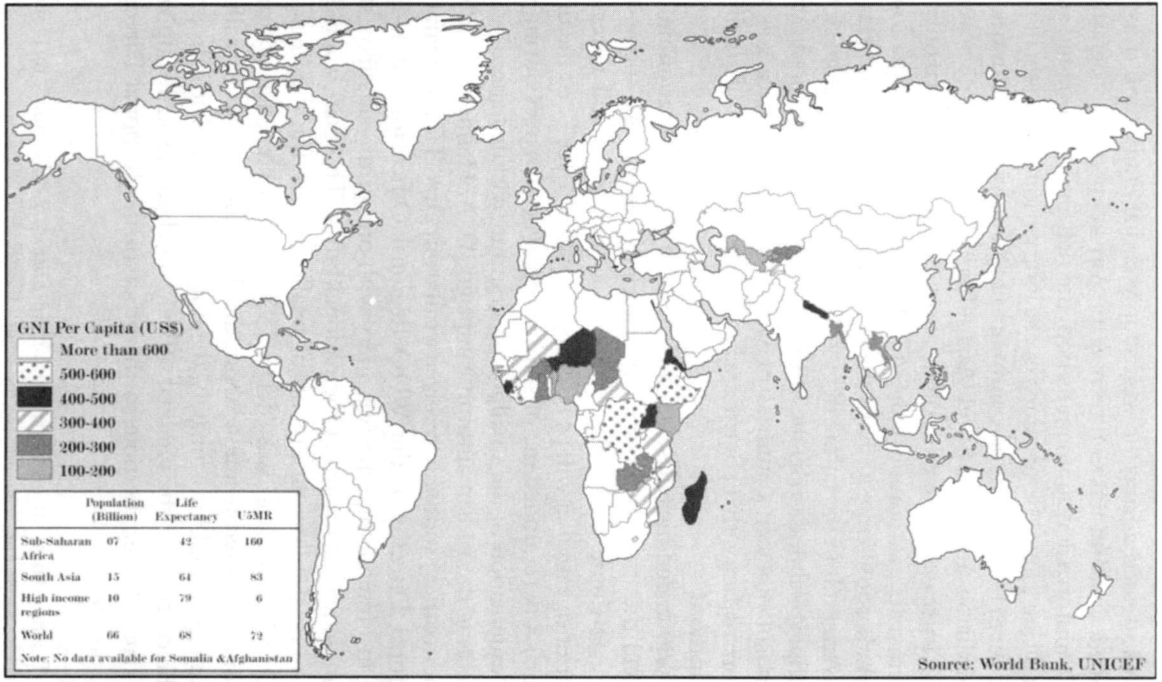

Source: Adapted from *Atlas of Global Development* (Washington, DC: World Bank, 2007), 128.

The Regional Director, on his part, indicated that the smallpox staff be fired for insubordination, and for not following the WHO rules. After listening to Gunaratne, Henderson politely but firmly replied, "He was right. The smallpox report had to be urgently handled without wasting time." Dr Gunaratne was silent for a while and then said, "You are right, he should fly to Nepal on the next flight." Often, when smallpox outbreaks were reported, our staff flew to the outbreak areas without following standard routine approval procedures.

In another, similar episode, smallpox staff at WHO Geneva were extremely busy during the last phase of the programme. There was much correspondence between the offices of the Director-General, the Assistant Director-General, the Division Director, and the Smallpox Eradication Unit chief, to deal with the correspondence from countries that had to be directed through the respective regional offices. One day, Ron Hauge, the administrative officer of the smallpox team at Geneva, carried a chair to the seventh floor of the WHO building and planted himself in front of the Director-General's office. I received a call from Halfdan Mahler, then Director-General, who asked me, "One of your staff is sitting in front of my door. What is he doing?" I answered, "These days we have an urgent draft proposal requiring your review and signature. He wants your approval as soon as possible. Hence he is sitting outside your door". I cannot recollect whether Hauge's method was effective or not, however, this was quite unusual behaviour for WHO staff at the time and even now.

Surveillance of Suspected Smallpox Cases in the Last Phase of the Programme

Laboratory certification of smallpox suspects was top priority. We often employed the WHO diplomatic pouch for dispatching smallpox specimens for testing from countries to Geneva and then to WHO collaborating laboratories (needless to say, paying utmost attention to necessary safety and secure packaging). No harm ever came from this practice.

Some field staff complained that preparing smallpox reports was too time consuming and took them away from the more important field work. I considered the response seriously and recommended, "You are right. We need only minimal reports, sufficient enough to assess the situation, such as the number and names of infected villages which had reported smallpox cases during the last week, with the number of cases and deaths." This worked well as such reports provided the required information on the priority containment actions.

In May, 1980, after the WHO had announced that smallpox had been eradicated, I often received many reporters at my Geneva office. They came from major press agencies—*Le Monde*, *the New York Times*, *Figaro*, *die Welt*, etc. They often asked, "Why did the programme succeed?" I replied, "Because we broke WHO rules". They smiled, thinking I was joking. It was partly true, though. I hope that readers will now understand the meaning behind the joke.

After the completion of the smallpox eradication programme successfully, I tried to convince other WHO health projects to take on the smallpox programme staff, from the headquarters, regional offices, and individual countries. They were after all rendered jobless once the smallpox menace had been dealt with! Surprisingly, I met stiff resistance. Many WHO project chiefs were reluctant to employ ex-smallpox programme staff as they were to some extent concerned about our working style, and that smallpox staff sometimes bent the rules. Of course, this was the exception rather than the rule. Generally speaking, at that time, it was prevailing health policy that the strengthening of basic health service take first priority instead of focusing on special disease control or eradication measures; and the concept of primary health care should be the tool. In fact, WHO's catch phrase was "Health For All", to celebrate the impending twenty-first century in 2000, using the tool of primary health care. Thus smallpox eradication, that addressed just one disease, was out of the prevailing mainstream in international public health at that time.

These anecdotes, except the last one, are the nice memories how smallpox eradication provided excellent teamwork towards achieving target zero. Even to this day, a few decades later, such mutual understanding is evident on many occasions.

22

Post-eradication Era: The First Three Decades and Future Perspectives

Vaccination Policies

In the 1970s, in the final phase of the programme, following the achievement of zero smallpox cases, many countries in North America, Europe and Japan discontinued their smallpox vaccination programmes, before the completion of global certification.[1] Within a few years, following the WA declaration of eradication in 1980, almost all countries had discontinued smallpox vaccination. The international vaccination certificate for international travellers was officially discontinued; WHO deleted all reference to smallpox from the International Health Regulation in 1981.

However, the tragic terrorist attacks in New York City on 11 September 2001, and the subsequent distribution of anthrax specimens in the United States through the postal system, caused considerable concern about the threat of bio terrorism, including whether the discontinuation of smallpox vaccination was wise.[2] Following these events, emergency vaccination of half a million security personnel was conducted, but was halted due to the unexpected occurrence of vaccination complications of the cardiovascular system, after only 40,000 vaccinations.[3] It was

1 I. Arita, "Farewell to Smallpox Vaccination", *International Symposium on Immunization: Development in Biological Standardization* 43, 283–96 (Basel: S. Karger, 1979).

2 N. Stevens and F. Gottron, "Anthrax in the Mail", in *Focus on Bioterrorism*, ed. G. T. Foster (New York: Nova Science Publisher, 2006), 39–42.

3 J. D. Grabenstein and W. Winkenwerder Jr, "US Military Smallpox Vaccination Program Experience", *The Journal of the American Medical Association* 289, no. 24, 2003, 3278–82.

eventually decided that a nation-wide vaccination campaign was not necessary. The cause of the complications is still under study since historically such vaccination reactions have been rare. [4]

Surveillance for Suspected Smallpox Cases

Since 1980, WHO has developed a good surveillance network called the Global Outbreak Alert and Response Network or GOARN (figure 22.1). In 2005, it also revised the International Health Regulations to improve disease surveillance. Over the years, smallpox cases have been routinely reported and investigated, with all reports turning out to be false or of diseases other than smallpox. It has been comparatively easy to conduct smallpox surveillance, as there is the advantage of a clear clinical picture of the disease, usually difficult to mistake.

During the last decade, there have also been cases reported of human monkeypox (see chapter 18) in the USA and DR Congo in Africa. On both occasions laboratories have confirmed the presence of the monkeypox virus. In the US, the virus was found in pets after being imported from Africa. There is a possibility that such cases may occur in other countries too. However, person-to-person transmission of monkeypox is difficult and the virus dies out. However, smallpox vaccination to prevent this disease is not recommended because the vaccine can cause side effects in some vaccinees, although it is effective to prevent transmission of the disease.

Variola Virus Stocks

In recent years, WHO has begun preparations to maintain an international smallpox vaccine stockpile, as was done during the

[4] J. Neff, J. Modlin and G.S. Birkhead, G. Poland, R. M. Robertson and K. Sepkowitz et al., "Monitoring the Safety of the Smallpox Vaccination Program in the United States: Report of the Joint Smallpox Vaccine Safety Working Group of the Advisory Committee on Immunization Practices and the Armed Forces Epidemiological Board", *Clinical Infectious Diseases* 46, supplement 3, 2008, S258–70.

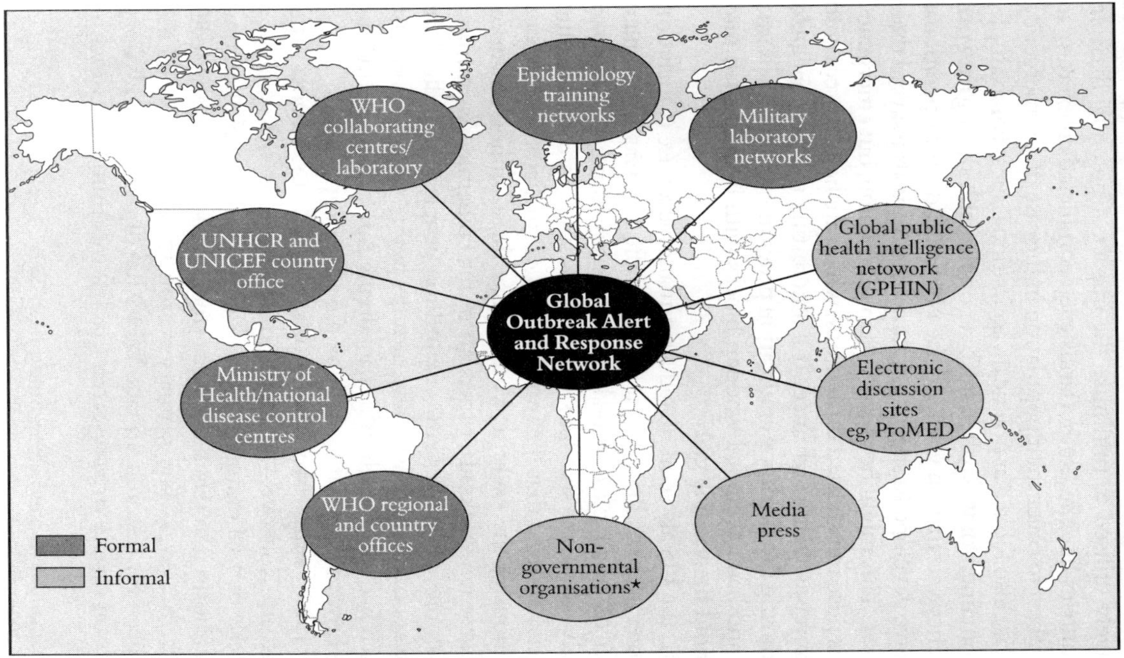

FIGURE 22.1 Global surveillance of communicable diseases

Note: * Including interested public as well as private health workers: In hindsight, they constructed the basic source of smallpox information.
Source: World Health Organization (adapted from a WHO original).

time of the smallpox eradication programme.[5] This is so that, in the event of smallpox outbreaks, the limited vaccine supply could be effectively utilised to minimise the impact of potential disaster. Some countries like the Netherlands even conducted an exercise to study how best to cover their population in the case of an emergency. The exercise also looked at practical vaccination issues. For example, vaccine containers or vials often fall over on the table during the rush of emergency vaccination work. In the Netherlands, the operational officers have developed a special container for the vials to avoid their tipping over. This might be regarded as a small thing, but emergency operations pose unexpected difficulties, which are better discovered during exercises well in advance. It is interesting to note that field workers during the smallpox eradication programme faced the same problem and had developed wooden blocks with holes drilled into them to hold the vaccine vials.

In 2001, the US also conducted a simulation exercise (Operation Dark Winter) on smallpox bio terrorism. The aim was to estimate the extent of smallpox outbreaks in the event someone were to deliberately release the smallpox virus. The results were astonishing. The exercise showed that the introduction of smallpox virus under the conditions of the exercise would cause three million smallpox cases in the seven weeks after the start of the epidemic. Assuming a case fatality rate of 33 per cent, one million people would die. The exercise was conducted just a few months before the 9/11 terrorist attack and it had a tremendous impact on the American government policy on how to cope with smallpox bio terrorism.[6]

Since 1983, only two laboratories—CDC in Atlanta and VECTOR in Koltsove—are authorised to store the smallpox virus. These two laboratories used to be the WHO collaborating centres, authorised to retain the virus stocks under the highest level of security measures. The primary reason to retain stocks of the virus has been for research. In fact, WHO has organised an advisory committee on variola virus research that has met numerous times to

[5] I. Arita, "Smallpox Vaccine and its Stockpile in 2005", *Lancet Infectious Diseases* 5, no. 10, 2005, 647–52.

[6] See "Dark Winter–Bioterrorism Simulation Exercise", http://www.csis.org/hs/darkwinter/.

guide the research to completion. The research is to include testing of the viability of the virus specimens retained, development of better prophylaxis and therapeutics, to update diagnostic assays, to update animal models, and to study various regulatory issues related to licensing new, improved smallpox vaccines. As member of the advisory committee, I often get to meet old colleagues who once were virologists from Vector. WHO has indeed provided us with a platform to meet and exchange comments on pertinent problems, which include need for further research, retention or destruction of the virus stocks and vaccine.

Variola Virus Stocks: The Risk Factors

The biggest risk factor for researchers when working with the variola virus is that they can get careless on safety measures while conducting their research. It is therefore useful to have the WHO advisory committee to review the balance between feasibility, practicability and usefulness of such studies versus the risk, especially in the current unsettled circumstances of world politics. In addition, there are unsubstantiated rumours that there are some unauthorised laboratories that still retain variola virus stocks, something acknowledged by the World Health Assembly (WHA) in its resolution WHA 60.1 in 2007 that "unknown stocks of live variola virus might exist".

Discussions on how to eliminate the risk of a deliberate smallpox virus release or escape through laboratory error have taken place among the international public health community, including the WHA and the implementation group of the Biological Weapons Convention (BWC). Following the Second World War, a few western nations recognised the dangers of biological warfare and began discussions that led to eventual development of the "Convention on the Prohibition of the Development, Production and Stockpiling of Bacteriological (Biological) and Toxin Weapons, and on their Destruction". The convention was signed in London, Moscow and Washington, DC on 10 April 1972. By 2005, the number of states party to the BWC grew to 155, along with sixteen signatory states. The convention's first article includes the following text:

"Each state party to this Convention undertakes never in any circumstances to develop, produce, stockpile or otherwise acquire or retain . . . [all types of biological and chemical weapons] . . ." . In my understanding, inclusion of the variola virus in the discussions of BWC is appropriate.[7]

In the last three decades since smallpox eradication, efforts have been made through international debate to destroy the remaining virus stocks. However, as far as I am aware, such proposals have not yet been agreed on. The latest decision by the 60th World Health Assembly, in 2007, in its resolution WHA 60.1, was to identify the required research subjects, with the WHO Director-General, and request to undertake a major review in 2010 of the results of the research undertaken or currently underway, and the plans and requirements for further essential research for public health purposes. The results of the review will be submitted to the WHA in 2011, which may reach global public consensus on the timing of the destruction of existing variola virus stocks.

According to the WHO World Health Report published in 2007, *A Safer Future: Global Public Health Security in the 21st Century*, "the greatest fear is that in the absence of global capacity to contain an outbreak rapidly, smallpox might re-establish endemicity, undoing one of public health's greatest achievements". The concern is legitimate if we consider globalisation and the rapidly developing global travel patterns, as well as the remaining areas of extreme poverty, such as found in some countries in sub-Saharan Africa. It will be difficult to rapidly vaccinate people, and to rapidly stop transmission in the event of smallpox cases being imported into such areas. The population density in and around the main cities in countries with high levels of poverty, an important criteria for smallpox transmission, is much higher today than it was during the time of the smallpox eradication work.[8] Whatever be the case, we should remember that since 1980, when WHO recommended the

[7] For more information on the BWC, see Mark Wheelis, Lajos Rózsa, and Malcolm Dando, eds., *Deadly Cultures, Biological Weapons since 1945* (Cambridge, MA: Harvard University Press, 2006).

[8] I. Arita, J. Wickett and F. Fenner, "Impact of Population Density on Immunization Programmes", *The Journal of Hygiene* 96, no. 3 1986, 459–66.

discontinuing of smallpox vaccination worldwide, the population not protected by smallpox vaccination has been constantly increasing. Those who were born in 1981, after smallpox vaccination was discontinued, will be 70 years old in 2050. This means that almost the entire world population will not have been vaccinated against smallpox if a case occurred. The disaster that could unfold would be unbearable. It would be self-explanatory that our human race has to develop decisive measure to avoid this potential catastrophe much earlier than the middle of this century.

How to Treat Variola Virus Stocks

Given below are my personal views on the subject of destroying/ retaining virus stocks in the collaborating laboratories.

Destruction of the virus

- **Advantage**: The completion of smallpox eradication. No risk of lab-associated smallpox infection as well as no risk of deliberate release of the virus.
- **Disadvantage**: Impossibile to conduct research requiring the live virus. Possible presence of hidden virus stocks.
- **Comments**: In case of smallpox return, the current technology is adequate to eliminate foci although there would be considerable hazards due to unpreparedness. Current studies such as new therapeutic substances, continued vaccine or diagnostic technology are not essential to be continued. Certainly, some would be good for some nations, but not needed from the global point of view. For instance, the treatment of smallpox patients would not be an effective method to cope with epidemics in poor nations such as those in Sub-Saharan Africa or South Asia. Note, the return of smallpox, if it occurred in Sub-Saharan Africa, would cause serious global epidemics. Thus, the research benefit is limited from the global point of view. The destruction of the virus stocks would be the rational conclusion.

Retainment of the virus stocks in WHO collaborating labs in USA and Russia.

- **Advantage**: Studies can continue with available virus stocks. These stocks are being kept under a good security system. If new studies need to be conducted, as their usefulness would emerge along with the development of new technology or epidemiological changes in the future, it would be possible to cope with such a situation. This includes emergence of new pathogens resembling variola in nature.
- **Disadvantage**: Risk of lab-associated smallpox infection cannot be eliminated despite all human efforts, even in the two labs mentioned above. National possession of the virus stocks, although at WHO-related centres, is viewed as politically inappropriate in the international community.
- **Comments**: The argument to continue research would appear to be weak, as mentioned above in case of the virus destruction. For the survival of humanity, disease eradication would be regarded as an unprecedented event in the history of evolution of biological species, as discussed by Darwin. From this point of view, it would be appropriate to keep a few representative samples of the variola virus in the safest place under strong UN supervision and security.

Conclusion

In a practical sense, destruction of the virus is recommended; however, from the view point of human evolution it would be appropriate to retain the virus at UN premises under the UN security system.This would help in two ways: (i) Minimise the risk of the return of smallpox; and (ii) sustain the availability of the virus if its use for research is justified by the UN. This would clearly demonstrate to any individual, group or nation that actions which increase the risk of the return of the smallpox virus must be regarded as amongst the most dangerous criminal acts for the human race. The smallpox eradication programme was successful only because the UN and the WHO conducted it. Why shouldn't the UN once again play the leading role to tackle this difficult and final issue?

A more comprehensive view on how to treat variola virus stocks will be discussed in the next chapter because we never know how the current progressing biological technology could play an important role to cope with the necessity to protect human species by sustaining the extinction of variola virus species in nature: for instance, see how over the last ten years the results of human genome research have influenced on basic biological research and basic medical research.[9]

[9] See "Science after the Sequence", *Nature*, 24 June 2010, 1000–1.

23

Research Topics in the Post-eradication Era

In the last three decades of the post-eradication period, while research activities have not attracted so much of the limelight in the global scientific community, critical initiatives have been undertaken to sustain the extinction of the variola virus on this planet. WHO has taken quiet leadership for the promotion of research in areas such as molecular biology of poxvirus, therapeutics and prophylaxis. Some practical aspects of these areas have already been touched upon in the previous chapters on vaccination policy, variola virus stocks and surveillance. In this chapter, some salient aspects of the research being conducted will be discussed within the context of preventing the return of smallpox. Some of the subjects are highly technical and evolving, and it is hoped that those who are interested would seek further information as needed.

Molecular Biology of Poxviruses

The complete genome of vaccinia virus (Copenhagen strain) [1] and smallpox variola major (Bangladesh 1975) [2], and attenuated vaccinia virus strains, LC16m0 and LC16m8 [3] were sequenced, indicating that the genome size of both viruses are about 190,000 base pairs. They

[1] S. J. Goebel, G. P. Johnson, M.E. Perkus, S. W. Davis, J. P. Winslow and E. Paoletti, "The Complete DNA Sequence of Vaccinia Virus", *Virology* 179, no. 1, 1990, 247–66, 517–63.

[2] R. F. Massung, L. I. Liu, J. Qi, J. C. Knight, T. E. Yuran and A. R. Kerlavage et al., "Analysis of the Complete Genome of Smallpox Variola Major Virus Strain Bangladesh-1975", *Virology* 201, no. 2, 1994, 215–40.

[3] S. Morikawa and T. Sakiyama, H. Hasegawa, M. Saijo, A. Maeda, and I. Kurane et al., "An Attenuated LC16m8 Smallpox Vaccine: Analysis of Full-genome Sequence and Induction of Immune Protection", *Virology* 79, no. 18, 2005, 11873–91.

are the largest sized among those of animal viruses and contrast to the 7,500 base pairs of the polio virus which can be now synthesised in a test tube.[4] Echard Wimmer, in his recent paper, commented that, at the time, it was immediately predicted that a similar method could be used to synthesise any virus including smallpox. Reviewing further the recent rapid development of synthetic technology, he proposed that "it is more urgent to develop new strategy in order to protect us from misuse by fostering open research in the broadest sense, not by restricting it".[5] Thus, creation of a variola virus is not far in the distant future, if it were desired. This observation needs to be taken seriously into consideration when we plan to destroy the variola virus stocks, because simple stock destruction may not be the solution. In addition, there is no assurance that stocks in the two WHO collaborating centres are the only ones in existence on this planet.

As discussed in chapter 22, I feel that perhaps only UN-approved facilities should keep the remaining specimens of the virus, under full security to be approved by the UN General Assembly, in technical consultation with the WHO. Decisions would then be highly influenced by sound political considerations in addition to technical recommendations of the WHO. Also, if certain research is required using the variola virus in the future, such work will have to be approved by the UN General Assembly. With this method, it would be possible for the global scientific community to prevent, or at least reduce the risk of, any negative consequences of research, such as synthesizing the smallpox virus.

J. G. Breman and D. A. Henderson have studied the epidemiology of monkeypox in recent years.[6] However, there has been a

[4] J. Cello, A.V. Paul and E. Wimmer, "Chemical Synthesis of Poliovirus cDNA: Generation of Infectious Virus in the Absence of Natural Template", *Science* 297, no, 5583, 2002, 1016–18.

[5] E. Wimmer, "The Test-tube Synthesis of a Chemical Called Poliovirus: The Simple Synthesis of a Virus has Far-reaching Societal Implications", *European Molecular Biology Organization Reports Reports* 7, 2006, S3–S9.

[6] J. G. Breman and D. A. Henderson, "Poxvirus Dilemmas: Monkeypox, Smallpox, and Biologic Terrorism", *New England Journal of Medicine*, 339, no. 8, 1998, 556–59.

proposal to set up a a surveillance system, assisted by WHO, for further study, including information on strain characteristics.[7] Monkeys may continue to be used as animal models for poxvirus studies, including human and variola virus infection. However, a word of caution: variola virus appears to be extremely host specific suggesting the difficulty to produce appropriate animal models. For instance, experience has shown that to infect monkeys and non-human primates, high titers of variola virus solution for intravenous injection have been used. Human monkeypox infection resembles human smallpox infection, but it is difficult to be transmitted from person to person. This means that a non-human primate cannot be a natural reservoir of smallpox. Thus, the extent to which a non-human primate may be used as a good animal model is unclear and needs considerable further study.

Research on the biological properties of variola virus in terms of its effect on animals is most desirable and necessary. In future, this information can be also used during research to evaluate the effectiveness of any prophylaxis and therapeutic drugs, which requires evaluation depending upon the situation of variola virus stocks and any possible risk of return of smallpox infection.

Therapeutic Substances

Research on therapeutics is important in the post-smallpox eradication era, especially in the circumstance where an unexpected terrorist attack using the smallpox virus would urgently require, among other things, a large number of persons to join response teams. Many of these persons would be unvaccinated. At the same time, it should be clearly understood that implementation of any curative measures to control smallpox epidemics would only be effective in countries where the developed health system is capable of fully employing the curative measures, which has limited efficacy when compared with prevention. Thus, the effectiveness of therapeutics is limited, although such studies do contribute to our understanding of how to control the transmission of introduced

[7] WHO Advisory Committee on Variola Virus Research, *Report of the 10th Meeting*, Geneva, Switzerland, 19–20 November 2008.

smallpox in industrialised countries, which could decrease possible exportation of smallpox to regions with limited health resources. A therapeutic substance may be used as needed to manage smallpox vaccine complications.

In the past few decades, several anti-viral drugs have become available, including Marboran[8], Cidofovir[9], VIG[10] and now ST-246.[11] The last one appears to be promising.[12] In general, it has proven difficult to carry out successful research on therapeutic substances, particularly with the limited resources available. Thus, we should have a good strategy in place, strongly assisted by the global scientific community, to meet research objectives, under WHO coordination. Otherwise, there is a risk that the level of support may decline.

Prophylaxis

It is self-explanatory that in the event of smallpox introduction, the smallpox vaccine must be the first and most effective tool to prevent its spread under any circumstance and in all geographic areas. Concern was expressed about the threat of the return of smallpox

[8] V. Stefanesco and R. Mihailesco, I. Spinu and S. Popa, "Study of the Action of N-methyl-isatin-beta-thiosemicarbazone (Marboran) and gamma-globulin on Vaccinia Virus Grown in Tissue Culture: Preliminary Note", *Archives of Roumaines de Pathologie Experimentales et de Microbiologie* 25, no. 3, 1966, 629–34.

[9] R. O. Baker and M. Bray, "Potential Antiviral Therapeutics for Smallpox, Monkeypox and other Orthopoxvirus Infections", *Antiviral Research* 57, no. 1–2, 2003, 13–23.

[10] V. A. Fulginiti and L. A. Winograd, M. Jackson and P. Ellis, "Therapy of Experimental Vaccinal Keratitis: Effect of Idoxuridine and VIG", *Archives of Ophthalmology* 74, no. 4, 1965, 539–44.

[11] G. Yang, D. C. Pevear, M. H. Davis, M. S. Collett, T. Bailey, and S. Rippen, et al., "An Orally Bioavailable Antipoxvirus Compound (ST-246) Inhibits Extracellular Virus Formation and Protects Mice from Lethal Orthopoxvirus Challenge," *Journal of Virology* 79, no. 20, 2005, 13139–49.

[12] WHO Advisory Committee on Variola Virus Research, *Report of the 10th Meeting*. Also see S. K. Smith, V. A. Olson, K. L. Karem, R. Jordan, D. E. Hruby, and I. K. Damon, "In Vitro Efficacy of ST246 Against Smallpox and Monkeypox", *Antimicrobial Agents and Chemotherapy* 53, no. 3, 1007–12.

endemicity by possible bio terrorism in the 2007 WHO annual report. Finding a safer and more effective preventive vaccine, with easy delivery methods, has been the main research target of the international scientific community. In this section we discuss some current research on improved smallpox vaccines.

During the post-eradication era, research on an improved vaccine has been an important topic. Many nations have developed vaccine stockpiles with conventional calf lymph vaccine—even though it is outdated in its production methods and can cause complications among vaccinees when inoculated, although seldom—a significant hazard in healthy populations.[13] However, this vaccine has assured effectiveness, important in case of use in an emergency. Further, calf lymph vaccine has a solid history of long-term storage, namely no reduction of potency for twenty years in storage conditions of –20° C.

Smallpox vaccines can be divided into three categories. The first category is the calf lymph vaccine, namely conventional vaccine with the advantages mentioned above. The second category is tissue culture vaccine. Acambis Inc., in partnership with Baxter, has supplied stockpiles of Vero-cell derived smallpox vaccine using NYBH strain and has supplied stockpile of that vaccine to the US government for emergency use in the country.[14]

Box 23.1 Virus attenuation

Live pathogens such as variola virus cannot be used for vaccines because of their virulence. Attenuation means to reduce or abolish the virulence of pathogens while keeping the capability of inducing a protective immune response against the pathogens. A general method to prepare an avirulent pathogen for vaccine use is to clone pathogens *in vitro* and then evaluate the virulence

[13] J. M. Lane, F. L. Ruben, E. Abrutyn, and J. D. Millar. "Deaths Attributable to Smallpox Vaccination, 1959 to 1966, and 1968", *The Journal of American Medical Association* 212, no. 3, 1970, 441–44.

[14] T. P. Monath, J. R. Caldwell and W. Mundt, "ACAM2000 Clonal Vero Cell Culture Vaccinia Virus (New York City Board of Health Strain): A Second-generation Smallpox Vaccine for Biological Defence", *International Journal of Infectious Diseases* 8, supplement 2, 2004, S31–44.

of a selected clone usually by inoculating it into experimental animals. An example is the selection of LC16m8 vaccine: it was selected in a cell culture based on the pock size marker on the chorioallantoic membrane of embryonated eggs and temperature sensitivity, and its virulence was evaluated by inoculating it into various experimental animals including monkeys. The pock marker characteristic of variola virus was used to identify the virus in patient specimens during the eradication programme. If the molecular mechanism of virulence is known, it is now theoretically possible to make an attenuated vaccine by molecular design.

The third category is attenuated vaccines. Since early last century, vigorous efforts have been made to derive a less pathogenic strain of vaccinia virus by serial passages of candidate strains in tissue culture. Strains tested included CV1 and CV-11 in the US. DIs and LC16m8 in Japan and modified vaccinia Ankara (MVA) in Germany. They have been discussed in detail in the Red Book.[15] None have proved sufficiently immunogenic to warrant further investigation except MVA and LC16m8. This MVA strain was developed by 572 serial passages of Ankara strain in chick embryo fibroblast. It greatly reduced pathogenicity to man and animals, and is a replication-incompetent virus. Its immunogenicity is currently under study.[16] While the MVA strain may come to be useful for special vaccinations, such as to immuno deficient individuals, here it would be worthwhile to further discuss the LC16m8 strain which may have the potential for being useful for wide-scale use for epidemic control or preventive measures.

15 Fenner et al., *Smallpox and its Eradication*.

16 I. Damon, *The WHO Collaborating Center for Smallpox and other Poxviruses at the Centers for Disease Control and Prevention Atlanta,* Report on Support for Development of Second and Third Generation Smallpox Vaccines, 2008; P. L. Earl, J. L. Americo, L. S. Wyatt, L. A. Eller, J. C. Whitbeck, and G. H. Cohen et al., "Immunogenicity of a Highly Attenuated MVA Smallpox Vaccine and Protection Against Monkeypox", *Nature* 428, no. 6979, 2004, 182–85; L. S. Wyatt, P. L. Earl, L. A. Eller and B. Moss, "Highly Attenuated Smallpox Vaccine Protects Mice with and without Immune Deficiencies Against Pathogenic Vaccinia Virus Challenge", *Proceedings of the National Academy of Sciences of the USA* 101, no. 13, 2004, 4590–95.

This section is contributed by Masanobu Sugimoto, a molecular biologist with considerable relevant research on the mechanism of attenuation of vaccine strains in Japan, as described below.[17]

Attenuated Vaccinia Virus Strain LC16m8 and Its Vaccine

Brief History of LC16m8

In the early 1970s, in an attempt to produce safer replication-competent vaccines, So Hashizume in Japan developed vaccinia LC16m8 strain from the Lister (Elstree) original strain, which had been commonly used for preparation of vaccines against smallpox worldwide in the WHO programme.[18] The LC16m8 strain vaccine is manufactured for the stockpile in Japan.

The important feature of the LC16 strain is a much lower neuro virulence in monkeys and rabbits than the parental Lister original strain or other vaccine strains used in the eradication programme (see figure 23.1).[19]

In 1975, the Smallpox Vaccination Research Committee sponsored by Japan's Ministry of Health and Welfare summarised in a report the following results of comparative studies of field trials with Lister, CV1-78, LC16mO and LC16m8 strains.[20]

[17] M. Sugimoto, K. Ohishi and S. Hashizume, "Properties of Attenuated Vaccinia Virus Strain LC16m8 Stockpiled Against Bioterrorism", in *Focus on Bioterrorism*, ed. George T. Foster (New York: Nova Science Publishers, 2006), 1–15.

[18] S. Hashizume, M. Morita, H. Yoshikawa, S. Suzuki, T. Arita, and T. Komatsu, et al., "Internal Symposium on Smallpox Vaccines, Bilthoven", *Symposia Series in Immunobiological Standization* 19, 1973, 325–31; S. Hashizume, H. Yoshikawa, M. Morita, and K. Suzuki, "Properties of Attenuated Mutant of vaccinia virus, LC16m8, Derived from Lister Strain" in *Vaccinia Virus as Vectors for Vaccine Antigens*, ed. G. V. Quinnan Jr (New York, Amsterdam, Oxford: Elsevier, 1985), 87–99.

[19] M. Morita, Y. Aoyama, M. Arita, H. Amano, H, Yoshizawa, and S. Hashizume et al., "Comparative Studies of Several Vaccinia Virus Strains by Intrathalamic Inoculation into Cynomolgus Monkeys", *Archives of Virology* 53, no. 3, 1977, 197–208.

[20] M. Yamaguchi, M. Kimura, and M. Hirayama, "Report of the National Smallpox Vaccination Research Committee: Study of Side Effects,

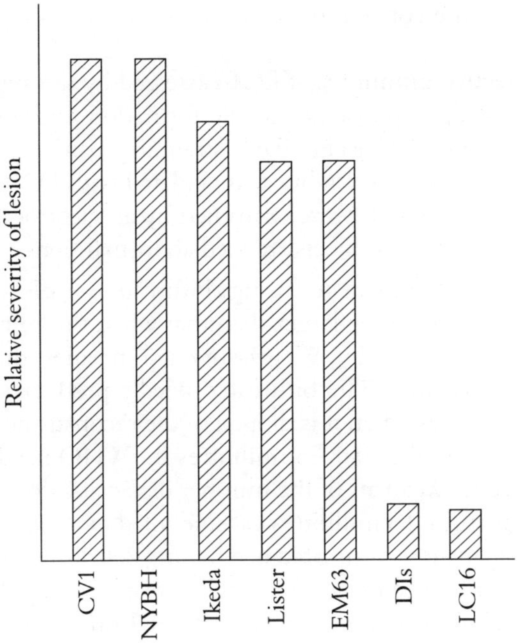

FIGURE 23.1 Severity of inflammatory lesions in the meninges and choroid plexus in monkeys

Note: The vertical axis indicates the relative severity of the lesion, and the vaccinia virus strains tested are shown on the horizontal axis. Monkeys were inoculated with 2 x 10^7 plaque-forming units of the vaccinia virus into one side of the thalamus.

Source: Based on "Morita et al.

1. No problematic side effects were observed among the 50,000 children inoculated with LC16m8 in 1974.
2. Among the 10,578 people who were vaccinated with the LC16m8 strain during 1973 and 1974, the rate of take was 95.1 per cent, the average incidence of fever was 7.7 per cent, the incidence of lymph node swelling was 12–13 per cent, and the mean diameter of induration was 6.1 mm.
3. The ability of LC16mO and LC16m8 to induce neutralising antibodies and hemagglutinin-inhibiting titers was comparable

Complications and Their Treatment", *Clinical Virology,* no. 3, 1975, 269–78.

to those by the conventional vaccine strains (CV-1 and Lister strains).

4. The protective immunity of LC16 assessed by the suppression of the primary response of pustule formation was comparable to the conventional vaccine Ikeda strain in Japan.
5. Brain waves of fifty-six subjects inoculated with LC16m8 at 14 days after inoculation were examined by an electroencephalograph. None of the subjects showed abnormal signs.

The vaccine can be inoculated using a bifurcated needle. However, the inoculum appears to be larger than that when the conventional vaccine was inoculated by WHO-supplied needles during the eradication programme. The bifurcated needle produced in Japan takes 0.005 millilitres when it is dipped in the reconstituted vaccine solution, as compared to 0.0025 millilitres for WHO needles. This makes a difference in terms of the number of vaccine doses that can be provided, namely 0.5 millilitres vaccine filled in a vial means 100 doses with the Japanese bifurcated needle, and 200 doses with WHO needles. The difference is significant when planning supplies.

Further, a clinical trial was recently carried out using LC16m8 vaccine in the Japan Self-Defense Forces. The proportions of takes in vaccinia-naive and previously vaccinated individuals were 1,443 of 1,529 (94.4 per cent) and 1,465 of 1,692 (86.6 per cent) respectively.[21] Seroconversion or an effective booster response among the individuals with take was elicited in 37 of 41 (90.2 per cent) vaccinia-naive participants and in 93 of 155 (60.0 per cent) previously vaccinated participants. The sample number was small, but the study did not find any cardiac complications among the vaccinees.[22]

[21] T. Saito, T. Fujii, Y. Kanatani, M. Saijo, S. Morikawa, H. Yokot, and N. Kuwabara, "Clinical and Immunological Response to Attenuated Tissue-cultured Smallpox Vaccine LC16m8", *Journal of American Medical Association* 309, no. 10, 2009, 1025–33.

[22] M. K. Arness, R. E. Eckart and S. S. Love, "Myopericarditis Following Smallpox Vaccination", *American Journal of Epidemiology* 160, 2004, 642–51.

The Study of the B5R Gene

A series of molecular-genetic studies of these temperature-sensitive strains by the study group headed by Sugimoto[23] in Japan identified a viral gene responsible for plaque size and the restriction of the host range, and ultimately for the attenuated characteristics of LC16m8 strain.

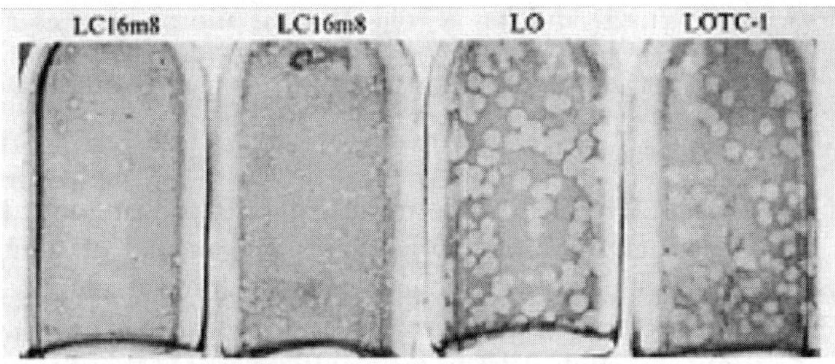

FIGURE 23.2 Plaques of LC16m8, LO and LOTC-1 formed in the monolayer of rabbit kidney cells

Note: LOTC-1 was made by introducing a DNA fragment of LO containing the *B5R* gene into LC16m8.

Source: Data cited from Takahashi-Nishimaki et al., 1987.

The results indicated that the gene was not only responsible for plaque size but also participates in the host range, that is, the ability to grow in Vero cells, and was named as *plaque size/host range* (*ps/hr*) gene (see figure 23.2). The *ps/hr* gene encodes a polypeptide of

[23] M. Sugimoto, A. Yasuda, K. Miki, M. Morita, K. Suzuki, and N. Uchida et al., "Gene Structures of Low-neurovirulent Vaccinia Virus LC16m0, LC16m8, and their Lister Original (LO) Strains", *Microbiology and Immunology* 29, no. 5, 1985, 421–28; F. Takahashi-Nishimaki, K. Suzuki, M. Morita, T. Maruyama, K. Miki, S. Hashizume, and M. Sugimoto, "Genetic Analysis of Vaccinia Virus Lister Strain and its Attenuated Mutant LC16m8: Production of Intermediate Variants by Homologous Recombination", *Journal of General Virology* 68, 1987, 2705–710; F. Takahashi-Nishimaki, S. Funahashi, K. Miki, S. Hashizume, and M. Sugimoto, "Regulation of Plaque Size and Host Range by a Vaccinia Virus Gene Related to Complement System Proteins", *Virology* 181, no. 1, 1991, 158–64.

317 amino acids related to the regulators of complement activation gene family of mammals. This *ps/hr* gene corresponded to the gene identified in the Copenhagen strain called *B5R* gene. The name *B5R* gene has now replaced the term *ps/hr* gene. The LC16m8 strain has a single nucleotide deletion that creates a termination codon at amino acid position 93 in the *B5R* envelope gene, resulting in a truncation of the B5R protein. The B5R protein is one of the envelope proteins of vaccinia viruses, and has a role in virus morphogenesis and dissemination, and as a target for neutralizing antibodies.

Potential Problems of LC16m8

The fact that LC16m8 has the truncated B5R protein, and that B5R is a neutralising antibody-inducing antigen of extracellular enveloped viruses, raises the concern that LC16m8 might have a defect in the protective immunity against smallpox.

Morikawa et al. studied the protective efficacies of LC16m8 against a lethal challenge with a highly pathogenic vaccinia virus, Western Reserve strain, in mice.[24] Vaccinated BALB/c mice were examined for survival rate and loss of body weight after intranasal inoculation with Western Reserve strain corresponding to ten times the dose of LD_{50} for these mice. Non-vaccinated mice died within nine days after the challenge with Western Reverse strain. In contrast, none of the mice vaccinated with LC16m8, LC16mO or LO died. Saijo et al. studied the effect of LC16m8 vaccine on the protection of monkeys from monkeypox.[25] Immunised monkeys showed no symptoms of monkeypox both in the intranasal-inoculation and subcutaneous-inoculation models, while non-immunised controls showed typical symptoms. LC16m8 strain exhibited a high rate of take and induced

[24] S. Morikawa, T. Sakiyama, H. Hasegawa, M. Saijo, A. Maeda, and I. Kurane, et al., "An Attenuated LC16m8 Smallpox Vaccine: Analysis of Full-genome Sequence and Induction of Immune Protection", *Journal of Virology* 79, no. 18, 2005, 11873–891.

[25] M. Saijo, Y. Ami, Y. Suzaki, N. Nagata, N. Iwata, and H. Hasegawa et al., "LC16m8 A Highly Attenuated Vaccinia Virus Vaccine Lacking Expression of the Membrane Protein B5R, Protects Monkeys from Monkeypox", *Journal of Virology* 80, no. 11, 2006, 5179–88.

a neutralising antibody response (the mean titer in terms of log 4). All these facts suggest that LC16m8 induces protective immunity against smallpox.

Notably, while the B5R protein induces neutralizing antibodies, many other proteins, including envelope proteins such as A33R, A34R and A56R, probably also have an important role in protection. Not only neutralising antibodies, but also cell-mediated immunity is considered to participate in protection against orthopoxviruses.

As for the management of vaccine manufacture, for instance, the introduction of a step comprising positive exclusion of large plaques from seed solutions and the use of only virus preparations after a few limited passages can cope effectively with the risk of mutation and reversion to virulence.[26]

In summary, LC16m8 vaccine would seem at present to be the best available attenuated vaccine for preparedness for control of smallpox if it returned, despite the fact that the vaccine lacks evidence from actual use of protecting humans from smallpox infection and this will continue to be the case in future. In the context of the international vaccine stock pile, the research subjects still to be studied, including this vaccine, need to be further reviewed by the WHO committee to decide the timing of variola virus destruction. Under the circumstances, it would be desirable to discuss whether anything more could be done. For instance, the neutralizing antibody produced by LC16m8 vaccine in humans should be made available for testing with variola virus antigen to ascertain whether it neutralizes the virus in comparison with other vaccinia virus of the first, second and third generation. The MVA vaccine was already tested in this way with favourable results. This may be done at WHO collaborating centres under WHO leadership.

In view of the last two meetings of the WHO Advisory Committee on Variola Virus Research[27] which referred to attenuated smallpox

[26] T. Kanehara, H. Yokote, K. Ohkuma, K. Miyamoto, T. Kumamaru, M. Kuranaga, T. Oka, A. Funatsu, and S. Morikawa, "Development of Consistent Manufacturing of High-purity LC16m8 Vaccine", The 6th Annual American Society Microbiology Biodefense and Emerging Diseases Research Meeting (Summary), Baltimore, Maryland, 2008.

[27] 29–30 November 2008 and 4–5 November 2009, in Geneva.

vaccine, LC16m8, the vaccine had advantages including the route of administration—the use of a bifurcated needle means that the vaccine is simple to give in the field—and that only one dose is needed (compared with two for vaccinia MVA). As in the smallpox immunisation programme, the visible take after vaccination means that it is easy to track those who have been vaccinated.

Conclusion

Research in the post-eradication era is handicapped by the non-availability of the eradicated smallpox virus as well as the uncertainty of research competence with surrogate animal models. Further, social, economic and political elements may reduce the efficacy of research. However, it is notable that so far every effort has been made, and will continue to be made, to reach useful conclusions from the research done so far. The current situation reflects the fact that unexpected and unavoidable difficulties may occur after any successful disease eradication effort, now and in the future. Hopefully, the discussion presented in this chapter will contribute to increased understanding of this issue for the reader.

In all aspects, especially the critical aspect of destroying or retaining vaiola virus stocks in the future, the WHO's coordinationand leadership will remain essential. My personal proposal is simple (as discussed in chapter 22)—a surveillance and containment strategy—and to stop research with variola virus in 2011 and retain representative strains in UN premises under strong supervision by the UN and WHO.

Epilogue

Placing Eradication in a Larger Context

The main lesson from the successful smallpox eradication programme is that when humans collaborate to achieve a common good despite differences of race, nationality, religion, background, culture, political system and unequal economic conditions, they can achieve great and lasting benefits for themselves and succeeding generations. Smallpox eradication was the result of the hard and effective work of all countries who worked for the programme, under leadership of an international organisation, the WHO. In particular, the world is deeply indebted to those individuals who worked under difficult, and at times life threatening, field conditions, not for monetary gain, but that future generations should be freed of the scourge of smallpox.

The smallpox eradication programme could not address two important issues: (a) what to do with the remaining variola virus stocks and (b) how to prevent the release of the virus from existing research laboratories or from unknown stocks of the virus elsewhere if they exist. These issues are not only technical in nature, but also political and therefore have to be dealt with tactfully.

There is always the worry that the virus may be used not just by terrorists, but also by nations in warfare. It is hoped that the destruction of the stocks in the WHO collaborating laboratories will take place in the future, when the currently WHO-approved research with variola virus is ended, perhaps in 2011. However, until then, there is no guarantee that, if there are several remaining stocks of the virus elsewhere in the world, the synthetic development of the virus could not take place. Thus, as discussed in chapters 22 and 23, my proposal is that the representative species of variola virus be kept at UN/WHO premises with strong security supervision. This treatment would give the clear message to the world that the stock of variola virus is only kept by the UN, the virtual parliament of man.[1] Also, we cannot exclude the possibility that we may need to further study the virus in the future. One never knows. I hope this would constantly provide a warning to those who wish to keep the virus for their own selfish purpose. Hopefully, further detailed discussions will be held by UN/WHO in due course, which would help prevent any catastrophic disaster in future. As discussed in chapter 22, action will be needed well before 2050 when the global population would become extensively susceptible to the smallpox infection if it were to occur.

Smallpox eradication resulted in several legacy programmes such as the Expanded Programme on Immunization (further developed to a programme for global immunization strategy), research and development of new vaccines, and effective surveillance and vaccination-based infectious diseases eradication efforts such as for polio and measles. Of course, the outcomes of these heroic enterprises remain to be seen. Although the current world situation would appear disappointing, as Joseph Stiglitz mentioned in his book *Globalization and its Discontent*, I believe the success of smallpox eradication could provide a silver lining to our hope.[2]

The victims of vaccine preventable diseases are most often infants and children under five years of age in the regions of extreme poverty. Why should children in such areas suffer from the misery of such easily preventable diseases? They are innocent and dependent on all of us for their health and future. According to John Rawls, an American political and moral philosopher, all of mankind is responsible for this misery. Its continuation should be declared unacceptable by us all.[3]

[1] P. Kennedy, *The Parliament of Man, the Past, Present, and Future of the United Nations* (New York: Random House, 2006).

[2] See chapter 2, "Broken Promises", in Joseph Stiglitz, *Globalization and Its Discontent* (London: Penguin, 2002).

[3] See chapter 2, "Outlaw States", in Noam Chomsky, *Failed States* (London: Penguin, 2006).

War and Peaceful Development

The smallpox eradication programme was completed successfully at the height of the Cold War. At the time, the only major upheavals in the world were the Biafra civil war in Nigeria in the late 1960s, which fortunately ended just before the intensified eradication work started; the Indo–Pakistan War during 1970–71; and the Ethiopia-Somalia war during 1976–77. The Indo–Pakistan War resulted in a massive reintroduction of smallpox into Bangladesh (previously East Pakistan), and caused a substantial delay in the Asian programme. The Ethiopia–Somalia war occurred in the Ogaden desert where hidden smallpox foci were smouldering in the border areas between these two countries. The result was that the last endemic smallpox case on earth occurred in this area.

These epidemics caused by wars could fortunately be controlled, thanks to the rapid and concerted global collaborative effort, under the leadership of WHO, which could well be considered a "Global Parliament for Health". Besides these wars, there were no other major obstacles in the way of the smallpox programme and the smallpox eradication work continued unhindered. I myself visited more than forty countries during the programme, working not only in the national capitals but also remote rural areas. In Mogadishu, Somalia, during the last operation in the Horn of Africa, I often walked alone to my hotel at midnight or two o'clock in the morning after a meeting. It was safe, a much different situation than today. There were exceptions, of course, and as mentioned before, many staff worked under very dangerous, even life threatening conditions. The three incidences when WHO smallpox officers were arrested by some armed groups in the Ogaden desert certainly caused us much worry. Thankfully, they were released soon afterwards.These were different times than today, with international and UN staff viewed in a different light.

We humans, since the pre-historic Pleistocene time about 100,000 years ago, have been experiencing a balance between parochialism and altruism. In other words, killing or reconciliation during the struggle for existence. The reason why humans have survived until now on this planet and will survive in future is because such survival tactics have been incorporated into our genes in the course of evolution. This is what Samuel Bowles, a behavioural science expert, said in *Nature*, 20 November 2008, while referring to the commemorations that were to take place around the 150th anniversary of the publication of Darwin's *On The Origin of Species*. Bowles noted that "parochialism and altruism act synergistically". Thus, if needed, humans may fight to eliminate or eradicate the enemy, or in other cases may settle on a strategy of compromise. Smallpox eradication succeeded during the Cold War, a period of compromise.

The length of the intensified smallpox eradication programme was relatively short: just thirteen years for eradication and certification. However, for those who worked for it, including me, it was a long and winding road. We succeeded in reaching the door as planned, but only with great luck. The genuine implication of disease eradication is not only a type of health measure; it is also a serious biological event by humans on this planet to cause the extinction of another biological species forever. We should not be complacent about such a significant event, so easy decisions on the road map of eradication should be avoided. The decision to eradicate a species requires judgement within the context of survival of human beings on this planet in future.

Bibliography

Alibek, Ken. *Biohazard*. UK: Arrow Books, 2000.

Arita, I., "The Control of Vaccine Quality in the Smallpox Eradication Programme". In *Symposia Series in Immuno-biological Standardization* 19, 1972, 78–87, International Symposium on Smallpox Vaccine, Bilthovern, The Netherlands, 11–13 October 1972, Basel: Karger 1973.

———. "Farewell to Smallpox Vaccination". *International Symposium on Immunization: Development in Biological Standardization*, 43, 283–96, Basel: S. Karger, 1979.

———. *Smallpox Eradication: Target Zero*. Japan: Mainichi Press, 1979.

———. "Are There Better Global Mechanisms for Formulating, Implementing, and Evaluating Eradiation Programs?" *Report of the Dahlem Workshop on the Eradication of Infectious Diseases*. Berlin, March 16–22, 177–86, New York: John Wiley & Sons, 1997.

———. "Smallpox Vaccine and its Stockpile in 2005". *Lancet Infectious Diseases* 5, no. 10, 2005, 647–52.

Arita, I., and D. A. Henderson. "Smallpox and Monkeypox in Non-Human Primates". *Bulletin of World Health Organization* 39, 1968, 277–83.

Arita, I., R. Gispen, S. S. Kalter, Lim Teong Wah, and S. S. Marennikova. "Outbreaks of Monkeypox and Serological Surveys in Non-human Primates". *Bulletin of the World Health Organization* 46, no. 5, 1972, 625–31.

Arita, I., J. Wickett, and F. Fenner. "Impact of Population Density on Immunization Programmes". *Journal of Hygiene* 96, 1986, 459–66.

Arness, M. K., R. E. Eckart, and S. S. Love. "Myopericarditis Following Smallpox Vaccination". *American Journal of Epidemiology* 160, 2004, 642–51.

Basu, R. N., Z. Jezek, and N. A. Ward. *The Eradication of Smallpox from India*. New Delhi: WHO South-East Asia Regional Office, 1979.

Baker, R. O., and M. Bray. "Potential Antiviral Therapeutics for Smallpox, Monkeypox and other Orthopoxvirus Infections". *Antiviral Research* 57, no. 1–2, 2003, 13–23.

Baxby, Derrick. *Smallpox Vaccine: Ahead of its Time*. Barkley, UK: The Jenner Museum, 2001.

Bhattacharya, Sanjoy. *Expunging Variola, The Control and Eradication of Smallpox in India, 1947–1977.* Hyderabad: Orient Longman, 2006.

Breman, J. G., and D. A. Henderson. "Poxvirus Dilemmas: Monkeypox, Smallpox, and Biologic Terrorism". *New England Journal of Medicine*. 339, no. 8 1998, 556–59.

Brilliant, L. *The Management of Smallpox Eradication in India*. Michigan: The University of Michigan Press, 1985.

Cello, J., A. V. Paul, and E. Wimmer. "Chemical Synthesis of Poliovirus cDNA: Generation of Infectious Virus in the Absence of Natural Template". *Science* 297, no. 5583, 2002, 1016–18.

Damon, I. *The WHO Collaborating Center for Smallpox and other Poxviruses at the Centers for Disease Control and Prevention Atlanta.* Report on Support for Development of Second and Third Generation Smallpox Vaccines, 2008.

Dumbell, K. R., and L. C. Archard. "Comparison of White Pock (h) Mutants of Monkeypox Virus with Parental Monkeypox and with Variola-like Viruses Isolated from Animals". *Nature* 286, no. 5768, 1980, 29–32.

Earl, P. L., J. L. Americo, L. S. Wyatt, L. A. Eller, J. C. Whitbeck, and G. H. Cohen et al. "Immunogenicity of a Highly Attenuated MVA Smallpox Vaccine and Protection Against Monkeypox". *Nature* 428, no. 6979, 2004, 182–85.

Esposito, J. J., J. H. Nakano, and J. F. Obijeski. "Can Variola-like Viruses be Derived from Monkeypox Virus? An Investigation

Based on DNA Mapping". *Bulletin of the World Health Organization* 63, 1985, 695–703.

Fenner, F., D. A. Henderson, I. Arita, Z. Jezek, and L. D. Ladnyi. *Smallpox and its Eradication*. Washington, DC: WHO, 1988.

Fulginiti, V. A., L. A. Winograd, M. Jackson, and P. Ellis, "Therapy of Experimental Vaccinal Keratitis. Effect of Idoxuridine and VIG". *Archives of Ophthalmology* 74, no. 4, 1965, 539–44.

Goebel, S. J., G. P. Johnson, M. E. Perkus, S. W. Davis, J. P. Winslow, and E. Paoletti. "The Complete DNA Sequence of Vaccinia Virus". *Virology* 179, no. 1, 1990, 247–66, 517–63.

Grabenstein, J. D., and W. Winkenwerder Jr. "US Military Smallpox Vaccination Program Experience". *The Journal of the American Medical Association* 289, no. 24, 2003, 3278–82.

Henderson, D. A. *Smallpox: The Death of a Disease*. New York: Prometheus Books, 2009.

Hashizume, S., M. Morita, H. Yoshikawa, S. Suzuki, T. Arita, and T. Komatsu et al. "Internal Symposium on Smallpox Vaccines, Bilthoven". *Symposia Series in Immunobiological Standization* 19, 1973, 325–31.

Hashizume, S., H. Yoshikawa, M. Morita, and K. Suzuki. "Properties of Attenuated Mutant of vaccinia virus, LC16m8, Derived from Lister Strain". In *Vaccinia Virus as Vectors for Vaccine Antigens*, ed. G. V. Quinnan Jr, 87–99. New York, Amsterdam, Oxford: Elsevier, 1985.

Henderson, R. H., and M. Yekpe. "Smallpox Transmission in Southern Dahomey: A Study of a Village Outbreak". *American Journal of Epidemiology* 90, no. 5, 1969, 423–28.

Heymann, D. L., M. V. Szczeniowski, and K. Esteves, "Re-emergence of Monkeypox in Africa: A Review of the Past Six Years". *British Medical Bulletin* 54, 1998, 693–702.

Hopkins, Donald R. *Princes and Peasants: Smallpox in History*. Chicago: University of Chicago Press, 1983.

Howard-Jones, Norman, "Thousand-year Scourge". *World Health*, February–March 1975, 4–11.

Jezek, Z., I. Arita, M. Mutombo, C. Dunn, J. H. Nakano, and M. Szczeniowski. "Four Generations of Probable Person-to-

Person Transmission of Human Monkeypox". *American Journal of Epidemiology*, 123, 1985, 1004–12

Jezek, Z., and F. Fenner. "Human Monkeypox". *Monographs in Virology* 17, 1988, 1–140.

Kanehara, T., H. Yokote, K. Ohkuma, K. Miyamoto, T. Kumamaru, M. Kuranaga, T. Oka, A. Funatsu, and S. Morikawa. "*Development of Consistent Manufacturing of High-purity LC16m8 Vaccine*". The 6th Annual American Society Microbiology Biodefense and Emerging Diseases Research Meeting (Summary), Baltimore, Maryland, 2008.

Lane, J. M., F. L. Ruben, J. M. Neff, and J. D. Millar. "Complications of Smallpox Vaccination, 1968". *New England Journal of Medicine* 281, no. 22, 1969, 1201–18.

Lane, J. M., F. L. Ruben, E. Abrutyn, and J. D. Millar. "Deaths Attributable to Smallpox Vaccination, 1959 to 1966, and 1968". *The Journal of American Medical Association* 212, no. 3, 1970, 441–44.

Von Magnus, P., E. K. Anderson, K. B. Peterson, and A. Birch-Anderson. "A Pox-like Disease in Cynomolgus Monkeys". *Acta Pathologica et Microbiologica Scandinavica* 46, 1959, 156–76.

Massung, R. F., L. I. Liu, J. Qi, J. C. Knight, T. E. Yuran, and A. R. Kerlavage et al. "Analysis of the Complete Genome of Smallpox Variola Major Virus Strain Bangladesh-1975". *Virology* 201, no. 2, 1994, 215–40.

Monath, T. P., J. R. Caldwell, and W. Mundt, "ACAM2000 Clonal Vero Cell Culture Vaccinia Virus (New York City Board of Health Strain): A Second-generation Smallpox Vaccine for Biological Defence". *International Journal of Infectious Diseases* 8, supplement 2, 2004, 31–44.

Morikawa, S., T. Sakiyama, H. Hasegawa, M. Saijo, A. Maeda, I. Kurane et al. "An Attenuated LC16m8 Smallpox Vaccine: Analysis of Full-genome Sequence and Induction of Immune Protection". *Virology* 79, no. 18, 2005, 11873–91.

Morita, M., Y. Aoyama, M. Arita, H. Amona, H, Yoshizawa, S. Hashizume et al. "Comparative Studies of Several Vaccinia

Virus Strains by Intrathalamic Inoculation into Cynomolgus Monkeys". *Archives of Virology* 53, no. 3, 1977, 197–208.

Mutombo, M. G., I. Arita, and Z. Jezek, "Human Monkeypox Transmitted by a Chimpanzee in a Tropical Rain Forest Area of Zaire". *Lancet* 321, issue 8327, 1983, 735–37.

Neff, J., J. Modlin, G. S. Birkhead, G. Poland, R. M. Robertson, and K. Sepkowitz et al. "Monitoring the Safety of the Smallpox Vaccination Program in the United States: Report of the Joint Smallpox Vaccine Safety Working Group of the Advisory Ccommittee on Immunization Practices and the Armed Forces Epidemiological Board". *Clinical Infectious Diseases* 46, supplement 3, 2008, S258–70.

Prothero, R. Mansell. *The Sixth Melville Memorial Lecture*. Evanston: Northwestern University Press, 1968.

Richardson, M., and K. Dumbell. "Comparisons of Monkeypox Viruses from Animal to Human Infections in Zaire". *Tropical and Geographical Medicine* 46, 1994, 327–29.

Saijo, M., Y. Ami, Y. Suzaki, N. Nagata, N. Iwata, H. Hasegawa et al. "LC16m8 A Highly Attenuated Vaccinia Virus Vaccine Lacking Expression of the Membrane Protein B5R, Protects Monkeys from Monkeypox". *Journal of Virology* 80, no. 11, 2006, 5179–88.

Saito, T., T. Fujii, Y. Kanatani, M. Saijo, S. Morikawa, H. Yokot, and N. Kuwabara. "Clinical and Immunological Response to Attenuated Tissue-cultured Smallpox Vaccine LC16m8". *Journal of American Medical Association* 309, no. 10, 2009, 1025–33.

Smith, S. K., V. A. Olson, K. L. Karem, R. Jordan, D. E. Hruby, and I. K. Damon. "In vitro Efficacy of ST246 Against Smallpox and Monkeypox". *Antimicrobial Agents and Chemotherapy* 53, no. 3, 1007–12.

Stevens, N., and F. Gottron. "Anthrax in the Mail". In *Focus on Bioterrorism*, ed. G. T. Foster, 39–42. New York: Nova Science Publisher, 2006.

Stefanesco, V., R. Mihailesco, I. Spinu, and S. Popa. "Study of the Action of N-methyl-isatin-beta-thiosemicarbazone (Marboran) and gamma-globulin on Vaccinia Virus Grown in Tissue

Culture. Preliminary Note". *Archives of Roumaines de Pathologie Experimentales et de Microbiologie* 25, no. 3, 1966, 629–34.

Sugimoto, M., K. Ohishi, and S. Hashizume. "Properties of Attenuated Vaccinia Virus Strain LC16m8 Stockpiled Against Bioterrorism". In *Focus on Bioterrorism*, ed. George T. Foster, 1–15. New York: Nova Science Publishers, 2006.

Sugimoto, M., A. Yasuda, K. Miki, M. Morita, K. Suzuki, and N. Uchida et al. "Gene Structures of Low-neurovirulent Vaccinia Virus LC16m0, LC16m8, and their Lister Original (LO) Strains". *Microbiology and Immunology* 29, no. 5, 1985, 421–28.

Takahashi-Nishimaki, F., K. Suzuki, M. Morita, T. Maruyama, K. Miki, S. Hashizume, and M. Sugimoto. "Genetic Analysis of Vaccinia Virus Lister Strain and its Attenuated Mutant LC16m8: Production of Intermediate Variants by Homologous Recombination". *Journal of General Virology* 68, pt 10, 1987, 2705–10.

Takahashi-Nishimaki, F., S. Funahashi, K. Miki, S. Hashizume, and M. Sugimoto. "Regulation of Plaque Size and Host Range by a Vaccinia Virus Gene Related to Complement System Proteins". *Virology* 181, no. 1, 1991, 158–64.

Wheelis, Mark, Lajos Rozsa, and Malcolm Dando, eds. *Deadly Cultures: Biological Weapons since 1945*. Cambridge, MA: Harvard University Press, 2006.

World Health Organization. *Final Report of the Global Commission for the Certification of Smallpox Eradication*. WHO, 1980.

World Health Organization. "Human Monkeypox in Kasai Oriental, Democratic Republic of the Congo (former Zaire): Preliminary Report of October 1997 Investigation". *The Weekly Epidemiological Rec*ord 72, 1997, 369–72.

World Health Organization Advisory Committee on Variola Virus Research. *Report of the 10th Meeting*. Geneva, Switzerland, 19–20 November 2008.

Wimmer, E. "The Test-tube Synthesis of a Chemical Called Poliovirus: The Simple Synthesis of a Virus has Far-reaching Societal Implications". *European Molecular Biology Organization Reports Reports* 7, 2006, S3–S9.

Wyatt, L. S., P. L. Earl, L. A. Eller, and B. Moss. "Highly Attenuated Smallpox Vaccine Protects Mice with and without Immune Deficiencies Against Pathogenic Vaccinia Virus Challenge". *Proceedings of the National Academy of Sciences of the USA* 101, no. 13, 2004, 4590–95.

Yamaguchi, M., M. Kimura, and M. Hirayama. "Report of the National Smallpox Vaccination Research Committee: Study of Side Effects, Complications and their Treatment". *Clinical Virology* 3, 1975, 269–78.

Yang, G., D. C. Pevear, M. H. Davis, M. S. Collett, T. Bailey, S. Rippen et al. "An Orally Bioavailable Antipoxvirus Compound (ST-246) Inhibits Extracellular Virus Formation and Protects Mice from Lethal Orthopoxvirus Challenge". *Journal of Virology* 79, no. 20, 2005, 13139–49.

Index

World Health and Smallpox Eradication

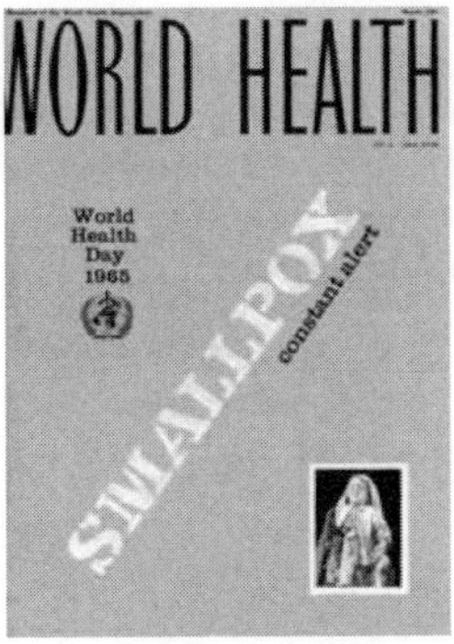

For the preparation (March 1965)

"The complete eradication of smallpox would not only rid the world of a disease which at present is a constant menace, but would also provide an example of what true international cooperation can achieve in a well defined and limited sphere. In the meantime, however, a constant alert against smallpox will have to be maintained throughout the world".

—Director-General, WHO,
World Health, March 1965

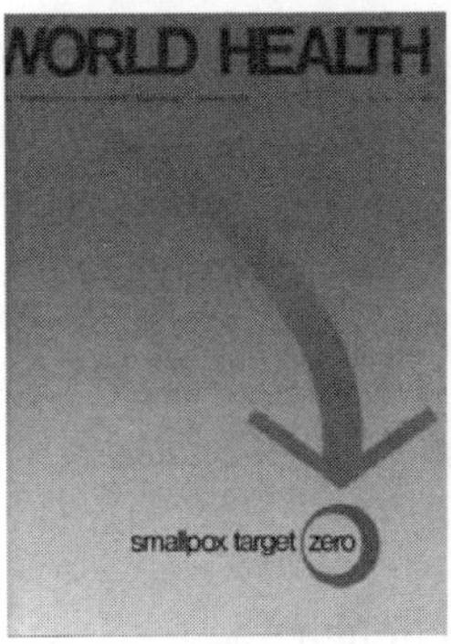

Target zero (October 1972)

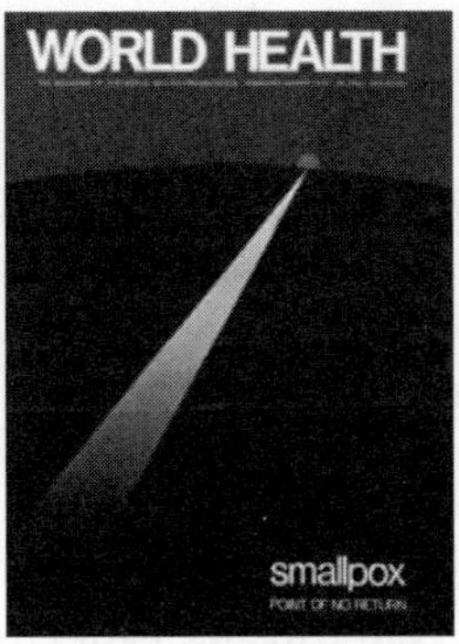

No return (March 1975)

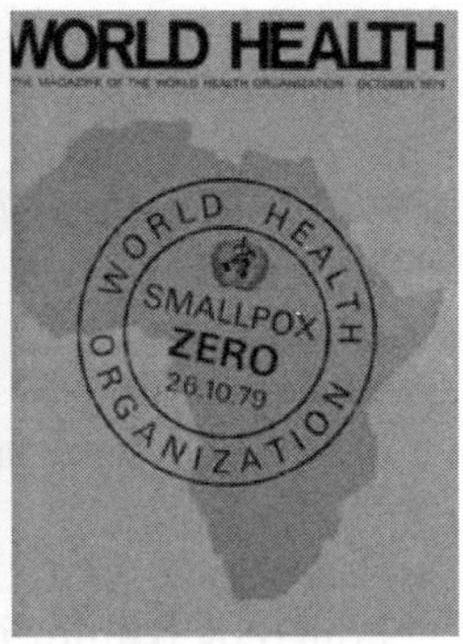

Africa free (October 1979)

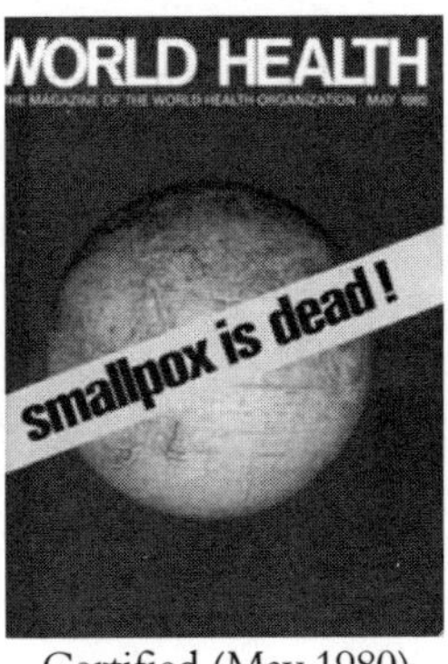

Certified (May 1980)

"Smallpox eradication is a sign, a token of what can be achieved in breaking out of the cycle of ill-health, disease and poverty. It comes as a glimpse into the future, an intimation of variable new order of things, in which world health, meaning health for the world, will have central significance in an upward spiral of economic and social progress".

— Director-General, WHO,
World Health, May 1980

Other titles in the NPSAH series

The Global Eradication of Smallpox
Edited by Sanjoy Bhattacharya and Sharon Messenger

Social Determinants of Health
Edited by Sanjoy Bhattacharya, Sharon Messenger and Caroline Overy

Low and Licentious Europeans
Harald Fischer-Tiné

Modern Medicine and International Aid
Susan Heydon

The Hospital System and Health Care
Margret Jones

From Western Medicine to Global Medicine
Edited by Mark Harrison, Margret Jones and Helen Sweet

Against Stigma
Edited by Balmurli Natrajan and Paul Greenough

Pathways of Empire
Ravi Ahuja

State of Vaccination
Atsuko Naono

Power, Knowledge, Medicine
Madhulika Banerjee

History of the Social Determinants of Health
Edited by Harold J. Cook, Sanjoy Bhattacharya and Anne Hardy

Taking Traditional Knowledge to the Market
Maarten Bode

Matters of Exchange
Harold J. Cook

Healing at the Borderland of Medicine and Religion
Michael H. Cohen

The Colonial City and the Challenge of Modernity
Sandip Hazareesingh

Refiguring Unani Tibb
Guy Attewell

27 Down
Edited by Ian J. Kerr

Decentring Empire
Edited by Durba Ghosh and Dane Kennedy

Expunging Variola
Sanjoy Bhattacharya

Reproductive Health in India
Edited by Sarah Hodges

Old Potions, New Bottles
Kavita Sivaramakrishnan

Fractured States
Sanjoy Bhattacharya, Mark Harrison and Michael Worboys

Health Policy in Britain's Model Colony
Margaret Jones

Travels to Europe
Simonti Sen

Science and National Consciousness in Bengal
J. Lourdusamy

Nature in the Global South
Edited by Paul Greenough and Anna L. Tsing

Civilising Natures
Kavita Philip

Inventing Global Ecology
Michael Lewis

Western Medicine and Public Health in Colonial Bombay
Mridula Ramanna

Woman and Empire
Indrani Sen

Situating Social History
Biswamoy Pati

Health, Medicine and Empire
Edited by Biswamoy Pati and Mark Harrison